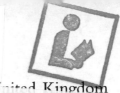
Gender and Health Care in the United Kingdom

GENDER AND HEALTH CARE IN THE UNITED KINGDOM

Exploring the Stereotypes

Bernadette C. Hayes
and
Pauline M. Prior

Consultant Editor: Jo Campling

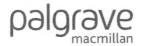

First published 2003 by
PALGRAVE MACMILLAN
Houndmills, Basingstoke, Hampshire RG21 6XS
and 175 Fifth Avenue, New York, N.Y. 10010
Companies and representatives throughout the world

PALGRAVE MACMILLAN is the global academic imprint of the Palgrave Macmillan division of St. Martin's Press, LLC and of Palgrave Macmillan Ltd. Macmillan® is a registered trademark in the United States, United Kingdom and other countries. Palgrave is a registered trademark in the European Union and other countries.

ISBN 0–333–77921–5

This book is printed on paper suitable for recycling and made from fully managed and sustained forest sources.

A catalogue record for this book is available from the British Library.

10   9   8   7   6   5   4   3   2   1
12   11   10   09   08   07   06   05   04   03

Printed in Great Britain by
J.W. Arrowsmith, Ltd, Bristol

This book is dedicated in gratitude to Frank L. Jones

Contents

vii

List of Figures

List of Tables

List of Boxes

Acknowledgements

The authors would like to thank a number of people whose help was invaluable in the preparation of this book. First, we would like to thank the staff of the Office for National Statistics and the General Register Office for Scotland, in particular Anne Blackwood, Beverley Busby and Julie Davey, as well as Dr Ciaran Acton, Research Fellow at Queen's University Belfast, for their valuable and much appreciated technical support. In addition, we would like to thank the British Academy, which provided a small grant to purchase census materials at the beginning of this project. We would like to thank especially those involved in the editorial process, in particular, Jo Campling (Consultant Editor), Houri Alavi and Jon Reed at Palgrave Macmillan and the very helpful referees. The usual disclaimer applies. On a more personal note, we would like to thank Dr Marysia Zalewski and Bobbie Hanvey for their support and encouragement.

Every effort has been made to contact all copyright-holders, but if any have been inadvertently omitted, the publishers will be happy to make the necessary arrangement at the first opportunity.

BERNADETTE C. HAYES
PAULINE M. PRIOR

List of Abbreviations

BMA	British Medical Association
DGH	District General Hospital
DoH	Department of Health
DHSS	Department of Health and Social Security
ECA	Epidemiologic Catchment Area Survey
EU	European Union
GHS	General Household Survey
GDP	Gross Domestic Product
GP	general practitioner
HALS	Health and Lifestyle Survey
HSE	Health Survey for England
IMR	infant mortality rate
NAO	National Audit Office
NCS	National Co-morbidity Study
NHI	National Health Insurance
NHS	National Health Service
NI	Northern Ireland
OECD	Organisation for Economic Cooperation and Development
OHE	Office of Health Economics
OPCS	Office for Population, Census and Surveys
ONS	Office for National Statistics
PCG	Primary Care Group
SMR	standardised mortality ratio
SSI	Social Services Inspectorate
UK	United Kingdom
USA	United States of America
WHO	World Health Organisation

1 Researching Gender and Health Care

Chapter outline

- Introduction
- Different perspectives adopted by researchers
- The problem of measuring health and illness
- Limited data sources for the study of health care in the UK
- The UK census reveals important new information
- An outline of the book

Introduction

The debate on the relationship between gender and health in Western Europe and in the USA has been ongoing since the early 1970s (for a review of the literature, see Hunt and Annandale, 1999; Lahelma *et al.*, 1999). This is particularly the case when physical health is considered. In the early years of the debate, it was generally accepted that two seemingly contradictory trends tend to operate at the same time. The first trend is that women consistently show high rates of morbidity – that is more self-reported illness and higher use of health services than men. The second and, seemingly, contradictory trend is that men have higher rates of mortality – on average, their life expectancy is five years shorter than that of women.

The relationship between gender and health attracted feminist scholars, whose work focused on the role of patriarchy in the medicalisation and control of the female body and mind (for discussion, see Macintyre *et al.*, 1996; Oakley, 1993; Showalter, 1987). The interest in women's health led to an explosion in studies on issues particular to women. In contrast, there were relatively few studies on men's health or, indeed, on comparisons between the health of men and women. In recent years, this situation has been remedied to some extent by the increasing number of national studies comparing the experiences of men and women in relation to specific health issues such as long term illness, mortality rates, and mental health (McDonough and Walters, 2001; Arber and Cooper, 1999; Lahelma *et al.*, 1999; Prior, 1999; Macintyre *et al.*, 1999). In addition, there is a smaller body of research on the impact of gender on the use of health services (Doyal, 1998; Foster, 1995; Kent *et al.*, 1995a; Morgan, 1980).

Current studies attempt to challenge preconceptions about the experience and expression of physical illness by men and women. This research shows conclusively that the simple generalisation summed up in the phrase 'women are sicker but men die quicker' (quoted in Lahelma *et al.*, 1999) is not always true. For example, when stages of the life-course are added, or when specific medical conditions are examined, the female excess in morbidity is sometimes present and sometimes not. One such study is that of Macintyre *et al.* (1996: 621) using two British data sources, the *West of Scotland Twenty 07 Study* and the *Health and Lifestyle Survey.* They found that:

> The direction and magnitude of sex differences in health vary according to the particular symptom or condition in question, and according to the phase of the life cycle. Female excess is only consistently found across the life span for the more psychological manifestations of distress, or is far less apparent, or reversed, for a number of physical symptoms and conditions.

Later in the 1990s, in a special collection of research articles on gender and health in the journal *Social Science and Medicine*, the complexity of the relationship was confirmed. For example, according to Lahelma *et al.* (1999), while the gender gap in mortality, or male–female differences in relation to life expectancy, is widening among young adults, it is declining among older adults. It is important to note, however, that although the gap is also large for injuries resulting from violence or accidents among young adults, it is small in relation to other conditions.

Other research points to the impact of the gender division of labour on health and on mortality rates. It does this by exploring the highly complex interaction between socio-economic position, health and gender, such as the inter-relationships between physical health and paid and unpaid work, employment and unemployment, and the impact of new patterns of work on the health of men and women (Courtenay, 2000; Doyal, 2000). Results from these British studies demonstrate that although more women than ever before are now in paid employment, they tend to have completely different work patterns from men in that they are more often in part-time and non-continuous employment, and they are also less likely to work in dangerous environments. As Busfield (2000: 81) comments:

> A higher percentage of women in the labour market than men have some form of white-collar work; they are concentrated in clerical, personal services, sales and shop work, where typically there are fewer mortality risks from pollution or injury.

Thus, women in the workforce do not seem to suffer from the same health disadvantages as men. In fact, overall, it seems that being in paid employment is 'good' for women's health – both physical and mental (see Annandale and Hunt, 2000; Bartley *et al.*, 1992).

The early research on gender and mental health has some similarities with that on physical health which considered the total population without consideration of age, social class, employment or marital status. On this simple level, it was clear that women predominated in all statistics on the reporting of mental illness and use of services (for reviews of this literature, see Prior, 1999; Busfield, 1996, 1994). From this it was inferred that women had more mental health problems than men. Later research, focusing on different age groups and on factors such as employment or social class, has pointed to a more complex relationship between gender and both the experience of a mental health problem and the use of mental health services (for full discussion see Chapter 7). This research demonstrates that although women still continue to be higher users of mental health services, men are becoming more visible, both nationally and cross-nationally, in studies of reported mental illness and in the use of institution-based services (Watkins and Callicutt, 1997; Payne, 1996, 1995; Robins and Regier, 1991).

Different ways of looking at gender and health

What is clear from these newer studies is that a much broader approach to the study of gender inequalities in health is now emerging. As with any other research area, different causal explanations are being offered for health differences in the male and female populations. As Lahelma *et al.* (1999: 89) argue: 'the pathways to health and illness include biological, psychological, behavioural and social determinants' and 'gender as a determinant of ill health is related to all four domains'. Because all of these factors are inter-related, it is sometimes difficult to come to conclusions on causation. Perhaps as Kawachi *et al.* (1999: 21) suggest, the focus on a particular cause is determined by the particular theoretical 'lens' – biomedical, psychosocial, epidemiological or socio-political – chosen by the researcher.

Box 1.1 Explanations for gender differences in health

- Biomedical
- Psychosocial
- Epidemiological
- Socio-political

Biomedical explanations focused originally on reproductive health. In particular, they sought to explain gender differences in health in terms of 'genetic, hormonal, anatomic or physiological differences between men and women' (Kawachi *et al.*, 1999: 21). While this approach was of importance in accounting for some gender differences in illness, it could not explain differences in morbidity and mortality in areas unrelated to the reproductive system. For example, the greater susceptibility of men to infectious disease mortality is attributed partly to genetic factors, but there is also evidence that gender differences in access to food and health care may be contributory factors. Another example is the higher rate of mortality from different forms of cancer among men. Although the gender difference can be explained to some extent by physiological and genetic factors, smoking behaviour and work patterns are also important (Waldron, 1997). Current studies generally acknowledge the limitations of the biomedical approach, although the ongoing research on genetics will add substantially to this debate (for discussion, see Conrad, 1997: Part 1).

Psychosocial explanations focus on male and female characteristics and identifications that make it easier for women than for men to report illnesses (particularly mental illnesses). According to this approach, gender differences in self-reported morbidity and health service use are a function of differences in help-seeking behaviour rather than any real differences in health status (see Courtenay, 2000; Macintyre *et al.*, 1999). Changing concepts of both masculinity and femininity in the late twentieth century in the United Kingdom (UK) might be expected to lead to a decrease in gender differences in morbidity statistics.

The third explanatory 'lens' – the epidemiological – focuses on risk factors and behavioural patterns affecting the health of groups of people. These include behaviours referred to by McQueen (1987) as the 'holy four' – eating, drinking, smoking and physical exercise – to which can be added sexual activity. In general, it has been found that men eat less healthily, smoke more and engage more often in high-risk behaviours than women do – leading to poorer health, especially among young men (for discussion, see Luck *et al.*, 2000; O'Dowd and Jewell, 1998). However, as with concepts of masculinity and femininity, these behaviours are changing. For example, British men are smoking less and British women smoking more than previously (DoH, 1998a; also see Chapter 4 for further discussion).

The fourth 'lens' referred to by Kawachi *et al.* (1999: 22) as the 'society and health lens', can also be termed the socio-political approach, which 'attempts to analyze the large-scale cultural, social, economic and political processes in society that produce differential health risks in women and men'. The importance of looking closely at socio-economic factors was shown in the work of Emslie *et al.* (1999), who found working conditions (not gender) to be the most important predictor of morbidity among men and women in full-time employment in Finland. The importance of socio-economic factors was confirmed in the work of Bartley *et al.* (1999) in England, who found that established measures of social inequality and of social class position were very good indicators of inequalities in self-rated health. The final excellent example of the importance of socio-economic status as a key explanatory variable in explaining differences in health outcomes is a study by Kawachi *et al.* (1999) of the relationship between the status of women and health indicators in the USA. Using a composite index of women's status (including political participation and economic position), the researchers found the relative status of women in different states in the USA to be highly co-related to mortality and to morbidity.

Two findings stand out in Kawachi *et al.*'s research. The first is that 'the higher the level of women's political participation, the lower their mortality rates' (p. 22). In other words, not only is women's health affected by their economic position, but also by their participation in social and political life. The second finding is that 'factors, which adversely affect women's economic security, also affect the material wellbeing of male members of the household to which women belong: including spouses, partners, sons and fathers' (p. 30). The researchers conclude from the study that the economic and political status of women in society has an impact not only on women but also on society as a whole. As Kawachi *et al.* (1999: 31) explain:

> Considered as a whole, a society that tolerates gender inequalities is also likely to be a more unhealthy place to live for both men and women, compared to a more egalitarian one.

In other words, while different theoretical models – biological, psychological, and behavioural – go some way in explaining gender inequalities in health, they need to be placed in the wider socio-political context of modern society.

Measuring health – the problem

Research on gender and health is complicated by the fact that there is little agreement on how health or illness should be conceptualised. As there are different theoretical models to account for gender inequalities in health so too there are competing conceptual approaches as to how health should actually be defined. To date, two competing models – the social model versus the medical model – have been proposed to measure health.

Box 1.2 Different models of health

- *Social model*
  A state of complete physical, mental and social well-being

- *Medical model*
  An absence of disease symptoms

The definition of health used by the World Health Organization (WHO, 1946) as 'a state of complete physical, mental and social well-being, and not merely the absence of disease or infirmity' is one that is almost impossible to measure. However, it is regarded by many as an ideal standard worth retaining. Basically, it represents a positive view of health, emphasising the relationship between health (physical and mental) and the individual's social environment. It is often styled the 'social model' of health. The alternative approach represents a rather negative view of health. It is sometimes called the 'medical model' due to its association with orthodox medicine. Health, in this view, is the absence of illness or disease. It is immediately obvious that this definition is much more useful to the researcher as it can be measured easily. Official statistics in the UK, as elsewhere, are based mainly on this definition – giving a picture of sickness rather than of health. As we have seen already, these statistics on mortality, morbidity and health service use form the basis for most of the current debates on gender and health.

Simple mortality rates are numbers of deaths calculated in terms of a defined population, for example, 'the infant mortality rate fell from 142 to 6.2 per 1,000 live births between 1901 and 1996 in the UK' (Baggott, 1998: 3). A more complex formula, based on the same principle, is used to compare death rates in different sections of the same population – standardised mortality ratios (SMRs). For example, SMRs are used in research on health and social class to examine inequalities in health: an SMR of under 100 indicates a lower than expected mortality rate – or better health – while an SMR of over 100 indicates a higher mortality rate – or worse health (for a full explanation of the concept and formula, see Baggott, 1998: 17). In research on gender and health, therefore, when the findings indicate higher mortality rates for men than for women in relation to a specific illness such as lung cancer, these have been calculated using SMRs.

Morbidity rates are calculations of illnesses suffered by people and are obtained in two different ways. Each involves the reporting of ill health – either to a researcher (self-reported morbidity surveys) or to a doctor or other health professional (surveys of health service use, including GP consultations). Research based on morbidity data, therefore, may tell more about patterns of reporting illness and accessing health services than it does about patterns of experiencing illness.

The difficulties inherent in measuring morbidity (illness) are particularly worrying when discussing gender and health. In the past, women have shown a greater tendency to report illness than men – whether this is to a health specialist (GP) or a researcher (for examples, see OPCS, 1996 and 1994). However, this appears to be changing. For example, research by Arber and Cooper (1999) on British men and women aged 60 years and over showed the opposite to be the case. They found that in situations where men and women had the same level of disability and where selected socio-economic factors were controlled, men were more likely to report poorer health. Other research also challenges the taken-for-granted assumption that women report their illnesses more easily than men. In a review of literature testing this assumption, Macintyre *et al.* (1996) argue that, although it may have been true in the past, there is little evidence in recent times to support it. Perhaps as concepts of masculinity (and of femininity) change, behaviour such as seeking help for a health problem might become more acceptable in the male world, thus restoring the gender balance (see Chapters 7–9 for further discussion in relation to mental health problems).

Help-seeking behaviour, of course, encompasses more than reporting the problem to a health professional. It also includes a willingness to comply with a given treatment regime – whether this be a stay in hospital or a course of medication. In the past, men were low users of health services – either in hospital or in the community – leading to the false conclusion that they were relatively healthy in comparison to women. However, in this book, we hope to challenge this view, adding to the arguments already voiced by Arber and Cooper (1999) and Macintyre *et al.* (1999). We will do this by introducing new information on one very important area of service use – bed occupancy in hospitals and social care facilities in the UK – and by discussing it in the light of existing literature on gender and health.

Although bed occupancy has not often been used in existing sociological literature as an indicator of health or illness, it has been used extensively as a measure of morbidity in medical research. One of its main advantages is that, in contrast to other morbidity measures, such as self-reported illness which is suscep tible to variation in question wording, bed occupancy is an objective measure of illness based on clinical medical judgements. This is not to deny the possibility of medical bias in diagnostic patterns, especially in relation to mental illness (see Part III for further discussion). Another advantage is that it has a high correlation with more established measures of health status. For example, research by Shapiro and Tate (1988) showed that poor self-assessed health is not only associated with early mortality but it is also a crucial predictor of institutionalisation. The final positive advantage of using bed occupancy as a measure of health and illness is its comparability over time, which makes an analysis of trends possible. However, this is not to say that it is a perfect measure. There is no doubt that the use of bed occupancy does not tell the full story on either health experiences or use of health services. For example, a key disadvantage of this approach is that, because it is based on the institutionalised population or individuals in the secondary care sector, it excludes from its estimations those using primary or community care services. It also excludes those who do not report their illness to any service provider but who might classify themselves as having an illness in a community survey on self-assessed health status. However, despite these limitations and as will be argued in this book, the use of bed occupancy as an indicator of health and illness provides a significant baseline for the examination of changing patterns not only in the institutionalised population – those using secondary care services – but also in the wider community served by the health care system – those using primary and community care services.

Data sources

Just as there are different theoretical approaches to the study of gender and health, so too there are different data sources on health and illness available to the research community. Most of the research on gender and physical health is focused either on self-reported morbidity or on mortality rates. Research on gender and mental health is focused less on self-reported morbidity and more on service use. For example, mortality statistics were used by the pioneering sociologist Walter Gove (1973) in his seminal analysis of the inter-relationship between gender, mortality and marital status. This relationship has been studied especially in relation to areas in which men have had higher mortality rates than women – for example, violent death, cancers and infectious diseases (for a review of the literature, see Waldron, 1997). One of the main reasons for the widespread use of mortality statistics in studies of gender and health is the availability of this information on a national and international level for men and women. Morbidity statistics, in contrast, are not so widely available in forms that are comparable over time and space, but they are increasingly being used in studies of gender and health.

In recent years in the UK, a number of surveys have emerged as valuable sources of information on health, most notably morbidity or illness, as it relates to other factors such as gender, income, ethnicity and age. These include the General Household Survey (GHS), the National Survey of Ethnic Minorities, the Health and Lifestyle Survey (HALS), the Health Survey for England (HSFE), the Disability Surveys, and the Survey of Psychiatric Morbidity (for a discussion on different data sources, see Roberts, 1992). For example, Arber (1997), Busfield (2000) and others have used the GHS to examine gender differences in reported illnesses. Likewise, Bartley *et al.* (1999) and Blaxter

(1990) have used the Health and Lifestyle Survey to examine the relationship between gender, class position and health behaviour. Other surveys, such as the Psychiatric Morbidity Survey (Meltzer *et al.*, 1995), have been used less widely to examine issues in relation to gender, though a similar study in the USA has been a valuable resource for debates on this topic (Robins and Regier, 1991).

These data sources, though excellent for the specific purposes for which they have been used, have important limitations which make them unsuitable for a study of gender patterns in health care throughout the UK. The first is a tendency to focus on only one part of the UK – usually England and Wales. The second is a lack of comparability over time – many of the surveys have not run for sufficiently long periods to allow for a comprehensive time-series analysis. The third is a tendency to omit the institutionalised population – individuals within residential health and social care facilities – from some of the more comprehensive health surveys. It was this lack of universal data on the use of health services in the UK, or the exclusion of the institutionalised population, that was the main catalyst for the research presented in this book.

Census data – the inclusion of the institutionalised population

While most of the discussions in this book draw on existing research findings, the arguments presented in the case studies, which form Parts II and III of the book, are based on previously non-analysed information derived from the UK census. In order to base our arguments on empirical data, we carried out a detailed investigation of census returns on bed occupancy in health and social care facilities in the UK – England, Wales, Scotland and Northern Ireland. Seven censuses were conducted throughout the UK during the twentieth century – 1921, 1931, 1951, 1961, 1971, 1981, 1991 in England, Wales and Scotland and 1926, 1937, 1951, 1961, 1971, 1981, 1991 in Northern Ireland – and all are included in the analyses. (For a discussion on the use of the census, see Dale and Marsh, 1993.) Census material prior to the 1920s is not included, as Northern Ireland was not established as a separate governmental entity within the UK until 1921 (Compton, 1993).

The data used in this book relate to the total population of individuals (excluding staff and visitors) who, on the night of the census, occupied beds in all officially designated health and social care facilities. These facilities include the complete range of providers (public, commercial and non-profit) in two distinct sectors. These are the health sector – consisting of all hospitals and nursing homes catering for people with physical or mental illness or disability – and the social care sector – consisting of residential facilities catering for older people and for people with physical disabilities or mental health problems. For the purposes of the discussion, a distinction is made between physical health care (usually known as 'general' health care) and mental health care. This was possible because all beds in the UK are designated as either one or the other.

The use of census data is particularly useful for a discussion on gender and health care for two main reasons. The first is the universality of the coverage. Everyone is counted – individuals in both private households and institutions. This is quite unlike the other empirical sources discussed earlier – such as household-based or other community-based surveys – which automatically exclude individuals in institutions. In other words, the census is the only comprehensive source of available information on the institutionalised population in the UK. The second useful characteristic of the census is that, unlike many other sources of data, this information is comparable over time and place. To quote Marsh (1993:5):

> The census has historically been the only reliable source of information about the institutional population, and can be used to construct a fascinating social history of the gradual changes in the numbers and types of total institutions in which people live.

This is not to suggest, however, that there are no problems involved in using census materials in a study of health or health care. The first major problem is the limited amount of information available. In contrast to people in private households, information on income, occupation and race is generally not gathered for people in institutions. This lack of information is particularly problematic in health research because of the importance of social class and ethnic origin in not only determining the experience of illness but also access to services. A second major limitation of census data is its lack of immediacy. Our case studies rely on data that end in 1991 because information from the 2001 census has not yet been released. This is of particular concern in this area of research in the light of the fact that there have been substantial changes in medical practice and health service provision during the 1990s. Despite these limitations, however, the analysis presented throughout the book, by including for the first time a detailed and comprehensive account of the institutionalised population, adds greatly to existing knowledge on the gendered use of health services in the UK.

Overview of the book

Part I provides a general overview of the nature and extent of health care provision with the UK. Laying the groundwork for the debates that follow, Chapter 2 presents a selective history of major developments in health and social care services in the UK, with particular reference to the gendered impact of many of these developments. Chapter 3 builds on this discussion by providing an empirical overview of this provision throughout the twentieth century. Again focusing on the gendered nature of health service use within the UK, it examines both primary and secondary service provision, as well as distinguishing between secondary care services in terms of those for the care and treatment of physical illness versus mental illness. The results suggest that, although women are higher users of both primary and secondary health care services than are men, within secondary care services the vast majority of both men and women are now concentrated in the physical care sector.

Part II focuses on gender differences in physical health. Divided into three chapters, it examines general trends in health service provision with particular reference to two specific stereotypes presented in current literature on gender and health. The two stereotypes are that people who are married are healthier than those who are not and, secondly, that older women are a financial burden on the NHS. More specifically, in Chapter 4, the gendered picture of sickness and of health service use is presented within the context of the general sociological arguments on causes of poor health. Building on this information, Chapters 5 and 6 adopt a case-study approach to assess stereotypical notions concerning the relationship between gender and physical health. Using census data on secondary care service use in both cases, while Chapter 5 focuses on the impact of marriage on health, Chapter 6 assesses the health care needs of older people, particularly women. In both cases, the stereotypes are confirmed. In terms of their use of secondary care services throughout the UK, married people are healthier than those who are not married, and the young are healthier than the old. It is important to note, however, that, while there is no difference between men and women in the health benefits of marriage, there are considerable gender differences in the health care needs of the older population. In other words, although the vast majority of older people continue to live independently in private households, older women are much higher users of secondary care services than are older men.

Part III concentrates on mental health. Again divided into three chapters, it explores general trends in the relationship between gender and mental health with specific reference to two stereotypical notions evident in current literature. These are that women have worse mental health than men and that young men are particularly shy when it comes to seeking help with their mental health problems. More specifically, the mental health statistics presented in Chapter 7 demonstrate clearly the gendered, albeit changing, nature of diagnosis and treatment of mental illness in the UK and elsewhere in the western world. As the data on secondary service use within the UK clearly shows, although women predominated in residential mental health facilities for most of the twentieth century, since 1991, men and women have become equal users of these services. Building on this information, Chapters 8 and 9 adopt a case-study approach to assess further stereotypical notions concerning the relationship between gender and mental health. Again using census data on secondary care service use in both cases, whereas Chapter 8 examines changing gender trends in the use of these services in England and Wales, Chapter 9 focuses on Northern Ireland. In both cases, the stereotypes are rejected. The results suggest that, whereas men are now higher users of these services than are women in England and Wales, it is young men – particularly those aged 15–24 years – who are increasingly finding their way into this type of care in Northern Ireland.

The final chapter of the book faces the future. The aim is to pose the questions confronting policy-makers in the first half of the twenty-first century in the light of the specific issues raised by a gendered analysis of health service use. A key factor which will be considered in this discussion is the future financial impact of the growing demand for health and social care services arising from an expanding population of older women. In particular, the choices available to future governments in meeting the needs of this population, such as the role of the private versus the public sector in social care provision, will be examined. Finally, the challenge inherent in mental health care provision in light of public fears concerning mental disorder, or the need for a safe society, will also be addressed. The importance of using a gender lens in relation to these issues and, indeed, to all health and social care planning, is highlighted throughout Chapter 10.

PART I
Health Care in the UK

2 A Historical Account

Chapter outline

- Introduction
- The early twentieth century: public health schemes put 'mothering' on trial
- The 1940s and 1950s: the increasing medicalisation of women's health
- The 1960s and 1970s: the gendered impact of community care
- The 1980s and 1990s: market forces are not gender neutral
- The twenty-first century: a new awareness of inequities (including gender inequities)
- Summary

Introduction

While much has been written on the history of the health care system in the UK, to date the impact of gender in relation to its development has rarely been assessed. Contrary to political rhetoric on the implicitly neutral nature of health care provision, it has been highly gendered in its impact. Irrespective of whether one considers the implementation of the first public health programme at the start of the twentieth century or the introduction of the National Health Service (NHS) in 1948, it is women, and not men, who have been the most adversely affected by developments in health care provision. With this understanding in mind

– of the differential impact on gender – this chapter provides an historical account of health care provision in the UK throughout the twentieth century.

Mothers in the spotlight

The Boer War, which took place just as the nineteenth century ended and the twentieth century began, brought to light the unhealthy state of many of the recruits (all men) who came forward for active military service. Fearing a downward trend in health in the population as a whole and of men in particular, the government immediately set up an Inter-Departmental Committee on Physical Deterioration. According to its report published in 1904, the individual was not to blame for his or her bad health because 'standards of health and morals were not genetically inherited' and recommended that 'environmental and behavioural changes could improve standards of health' (Jones, 1994: 23). This was a laudable sentiment. The resulting campaign, however, seemed to place the blame on 'bad mothering'. Alongside the distribution depots for 'pure' milk that opened throughout the country, there was an advisory service on child-bearing and child-rearing, aimed at developing 'good mothering' skills among young women.

Protests from the women's movement and the Fabian Society that this assumption was false fell on deaf ears. They argued that it was differences in social class and geographic location and not 'bad mothering' which accounted for differences in health status and, thus, that these changes alone were insufficient. Basing their evidence on a number of studies, such as Seebohm Rowntree's study of poverty in York in 1901, the protestors argued that economic and social improvements (including better housing) were an essential part of any public health programme. The need for state intervention to improve social conditions was also echoed by social reformers like Sydney and Beatrice Webb, who called for a collective response to poverty and inequality in the Minority Report of the Royal Commission on the Poor Law in 1904. However, in spite of the fact that a number of eminent people highlighted the link between poor health and poverty, health improvement schemes were narrowly focused on specific health problems and groups of people. For example, still focusing on children, school meals service was introduced in 1906 and a school medical service in 1907. These services, however, served only to mask the appalling physical conditions within which many families lived.

As it happened, changes in the wider policy environment had an even greater effect on health than these specific programmes, and all were highly gendered in their impact. The system of National Health Insurance, introduced by the Liberal Government in 1911, meant that manual workers on the lowest incomes (those earning less than £2 per week) had free health insurance, entitling them to free GP services and free drugs, sickness benefit and maternity and sanatorium benefits. The scheme was small to begin with, but it expanded gradually both in terms of the population covered and the benefits offered. By 1939, approximately 43 per cent of the population was covered by NHI and 90 per cent of GPs participated in it (for discussion, see Baggott, 1998: 88; Jones, 1994: 26–7; Allsop, 1984: 18). There is no doubt that the introduction of NHI was one of the most important developments in health policy in the early years of the twentieth century because it incorporated the principle of collective responsibility for individual health needs. However, it was deeply flawed. It excluded those who were not employed (including dependent family members), which meant that, far from being universal, it provided health protection for very few women and excluded children completely.

In spite of the gender bias in the NHI scheme and the faulty focus of public health policies during the first two decades of the century, there was a great improvement in health during this period. This was shown, for example, in a decrease in infant mortality rates (IMR). The IMR in Britain dropped from 154 deaths per 1,000 live births in 1900, to 105 per 1,000 in 1916, and to 80 per 1,000 in 1920 (Jones, 1994: 25). This improvement is attributed to a combination of factors, including a general upturn in the standard of living, the availability of clean milk, better sanitation and special medical attention for premature babies. However, other indicators of health, such as illnesses among the adult male population, were not so positive, and specific health problems continued to be highlighted throughout the First World War (1914–18).

One of the most glaring problems highlighted by the war, however, was the lack of co-ordination between the different components of the health system – hospital services, community health services and public health programmes. In an effort to resolve some of these problems and to move the health agenda forward, a Ministry of Health was established in 1919. The Ministry inherited a mixture of public and private provision with no obvious structure. The private sector, which provided the majority of general health care beds (Allsop, 1984: 25), was involved both in hospitals and in community health and welfare schemes. Though called 'the private sector', it was made up mostly of non-profit organisations and was most famous for voluntary hospitals, many of which had already been in existence for over a hundred years. However, the sector was in financial difficulties due to the withdrawal of funding by wealthy philanthropists and charitable organisations. This source of revenue had all but dried up by the 1930s and subsequently had to be replaced by an increasing reliance on patient fees paid either directly by the individual or by his or her health insurance club or friendly society (see Baggott, 1998: 86). In contrast, public sector hospitals and welfare homes, with their roots in the hated Poor Law, were becoming more acceptable to the public as a source of health care provision by the 1930s. A key factor in facilitating this development was the abolition of the Poor Law Board in 1929 and the subsequent transfer of all Poor Law institutions to local authorities, although its negative legacy did not disappear completely until after the introduction of a free health service in 1948.

The written histories of the health services for the inter-war period provide very little information on the gender of the population using these hospitals or welfare homes. We can conjecture that some hospitals catered specifically for women, for example, the maternity hospitals, run mostly within the voluntary sector. We might also conjecture that because women predominated in the older population (although not to the same extent as currently) they might also predominate in hospitals and welfare homes. However, as we shall see later in this book, this did not translate into an over-representation of women in these facilities. Contrary to expectations, it was men, and not women, who formed the majority in this population during the 1920s and 1930s (see Chapter 4).

The NHS – the increasing role of medicine in the lives of women

As the 1930s drew to a close, the health service system was at crisis point. Voluntary hospitals struggled to stay in existence as charity funds dwindled. Local authority hospitals and welfare homes faced increasing burdens of care as the number of people in poverty increased due to the economic depression. The NHI scheme failed to protect thousands of vulnerable people (mostly men with dependent families) who lost their jobs in the inter-war years (see Baggott, 1998: 90). Finally, public health pro-grammes failed to solve inequalities in health. As the Second World War approached, there was a growing conviction that only a radical shake-up of the health services system, with strong direction and adequate funding from central government, would reverse the downward trend in the health of the nation.

The solution came in the introduction of the NHS in 1948, which introduced a new structure – a tripartite system separat-ing hospitals, GP services and local authority services (commu-nity and public health) – for the health services. For the first time ever, all hospitals came under one administrative umbrella – though the teaching hospitals retained a privileged position in relation to the others. Thus, theoretically, at least, it would now be possible to plan a hospital service within the context of an overall health strategy. However, the delivery of this service would come with a large price tag. From the beginning, the NHS cost much more than anticipated. This was due partly to the poor state of inherited services (particularly hospitals) and partly to the increase in demand for services and in numbers of staff. During the late 1940s and early 1950s, managers were under strict instructions not to incur any unnecessary capital costs by plan-ning improvements or new projects (see Baggott, 1998: 98; Jones, 1994: 121). In spite of this warning, however, bed numbers in hospitals and care homes continued to rise during this period (see Chapter 3).

By the mid 1950s, it was clear that extra capital expenditure was needed to bring hospitals into line with developments in medical practice. However, the escalating costs of the NHS were causing grave political concern, so that, in spite of the recom-mendations of the Guillebaud Committee (HMSO, 1956), the major strategic document on proposed hospital development – the 1962 Hospital Plan – did not allow for expansion in bed numbers:

> The Plan envisaged a reduction in beds in most specialisms: acute medicine from 3.9 per 1,000 to 3.3; mental illness from 3.3 to 1.8 per 1,000; . . . and the number of maternity beds was to be increased from 0.48 to 0.58 per 1,000 . . . The Plan proposed a massive new investment by building 90 new hospitals and modernising others. (Allsop, 1984: 55)

This kind of forward planning for health services that would have fewer beds and shorter hospital stays could not have happened without the scientific advances that had taken place. The appearance of new 'wonder drugs' in almost every field of medicine was a feature of the 1950s and 1960s, as was the increasing medicalisation of conditions not previously treated in hospitals.

This increasing medicalisation of conditions had major repercussions as far as women's health was concerned. For the first time, almost every aspect of women's health became a target for the growing health industry. One such example was the increase in maternity beds envisaged in the 1962 Hospital Plan and welcomed by British women, as the preference for hospital-birth rather than home-birth became the norm. Another example was the growth in surgical interventions for women's health problems – hysterectomies, Caesarean sections and mastectomies. In the fifteen years between 1968 and 1983, the proportion of babies born by Caesarean section rose by 380 per cent in the USA, by 300 per cent in the Netherlands and by 250 per cent in Britain (Doyal, 1995: 138). Most people viewed this as progress. It would be a few years before the public heard the voices of feminists such as Mary Daly, Lesley Doyal and Ann Oakley, who questioned the increasing role of medicine in the lives of women (see Oakley, 1984; Doyal, 1979; Daly, 1984).

It took a tragic event in the 1960s to awaken the British population to the possible negative effects of modern medicine. Due to inadequate research and even more inadequate government monitoring of medical drugs, thalidomide had been given to pregnant women, resulting in the birth of a number of babies with shortened arms or legs. As a result of this scandal, which shocked a nation unused to questioning medical practice or expertise, the government introduced tighter controls and people became more aware of the fact that drug treatment was not a panacea for all ills. However, the healthy scepticism that emerged from this scandal did not halt the further medicalisation of women's health issues, which led to women's increasing presence in hospital beds during the 1950s and 1960s throughout the UK (see Chapter 4). On a more positive note, neither did it stop the drugs revolution in mental health care, a revolution that facilitated a radical change in patterns of care provision.

Community care – an increasing burden for women

> There they stand, majestic, imperious, brooded over by the gigantic water-tower and chimney combined, rising unmistakable and daunting out of the country-side, the asylums which our forefathers built with such solidity. (Powell, 1961)

Enoch Powell, Minister for Health, signalled the demise of the large Victorian mental hospital in this famous 'water-tower' speech. Part of the 1962 Hospital Plan for the new district general hospitals (DGHs) was that they would include some mental health beds and geriatric beds alongside acute medicine and that, eventually, there would be no need for the specialist mental hospital or geriatric institution. However, it took longer than envisaged to de-institutionalise the thousands of people in long-term care for mental illness, learning disability and physical disability. To add to the problem, the number of older people (particularly women) requiring long-term care was increasing rather than decreasing because of the ageing population and the increasing gender difference in life expectancy. In addition, the number of working-age women available to act as carers was starting to decrease, due to the increasing participation of women in employment and to changing views on the role of women in society. The job of unpaid and unrecognised 'carer' could no longer be taken for granted. As one might expect, therefore, the impetus for the proposed transfer of long-stay patients into the community did not come from the existing (predominantly female) population of carers. Rather, it came from a number of professional and academic sources on both sides of the Atlantic, and was welcomed by health research planners and politicians who were looking for a rationale to reduce hospital beds.

Increasing revelations of poor services for many people in long-term care, concerns over funding and ensuring value for public money, and the general dissatisfaction with the organisational structure of the 1948 NHS, however, led to its re-organisation in 1974 (for discussion, see Ham, 1999: 22; Baggott, 1998: 100; Allsop, 1984: 124). The intention was to provide structures and financial incentives to health authorities and social services departments to co-operate in a more integrated approach to care for all client groups (especially older people) and to speed up the transfer of long-term care from the hospital to the community. At least as far as the curtailment in the growth in health and social care beds was concerned, this strategy appeared to be highly successful. Occupied-bed numbers in the UK dropped dramatically throughout the 1970s (see Chapter 3). However, while some of the reduction might be attributed to policy initiatives such as those referred to above, it is much more likely that the main impetus came from changes in medical practice, or the move to day-surgery and day-treatment. This phenomenon that began in the late 1970s continues to change the pattern of bed occupancy within health care today.

It is important to note, however, that, unlike discussions on the health services during the first half of the twentieth century, accounts of later decades show an increasing awareness of the gendered impact of particular developments (for discussion, see Doyal, 1998). By the end of the 1970s, it was generally accepted that the health of the nation was improving on a general level – when considered in terms of life expectancy, infant mortality rates and mortality rates from diseases such as TB, which had been rampant earlier in the century. However, there was also an emerging body of evidence on inequalities in health, mainly in relation to gender, income and geographical area, but also relating to other factors such as ethnicity and age (Townsend et al., 1992; Mechanic, 1978; Gove, 1973).

On the question of gender, research findings consistently pointed to higher rates of mortality for men for most of the major illnesses, leading to an increasing gender gap in life expectancy. In relation to women, it was accepted that they had higher rates of morbidity as shown in higher rates of health service use and of reported illness (for discussion, see Jones, 1994). At this point in time, however, there were very few voices questioning why these patterns prevailed, and a low level of consciousness of the NHS as anything but a gender-neutral system of care. However, as we saw earlier, this was about to change as feminist writers highlighted the patriarchal nature of the British health care system in which most of the decision-makers (managers and senior doctors) were men, and most of the caring staff (nurses, speech therapists, occupational therapists and chiropodists) and most of the patients were women (Doyal, 1979; Oakley, 1984).

Thatcherism – a retreat from universal health care

When the Conservative Party came to power in 1979, few could have envisaged the impact of the policies to be introduced throughout the public sector in the 1980s and early 1990s. Influenced by the political philosophy of the New Right, the Conservative Government under two Prime Ministers, Margaret Thatcher and John Major, made radical changes to the health service system throughout the UK, changes that have survived into the twenty-first century under a Labour Government. As Baggott (1998: 102) points out, the philosophy of the New Right was not a coherent doctrine but rather a number of inter-related dogmas. These included a commitment to individual responsibility and choice, to a limited though strong state and, finally, to a free market economy. The Thatcher era is associated with policies to deregulate the economy and to introduce market principles to the public sector (for discussion, see Green, 1987).

These priorities can be seen clearly in the changes introduced in the health services in the 1980s and 1990s – changes that came to be known collectively as 'the NHS reforms'. The health service system throughout the UK was facing a number of difficulties at the end of the 1970s – funding shortages, industrial action and internal communication problems. Having sought advice from British businessman Sir Roy Griffiths and American health economist Alain Enthoven, the Conservative Government began a programme of reform in the mid 1980s, which radically changed the delivery of health and social care services throughout the UK. The two most significant developments in terms of impact on the shape of the service sector were, first, the introduction of legal structures enabling publicly funded hospitals to become quasi-businesses (Trusts) in a market providing health services, and, second, the acceptance of a 'mixed economy of care' in the provision of health and social care services. As a consequence of the latter, there was an expansion of private providers in many specialties, but especially in that of long-term care of older people, the majority of whom were women.

These two developments had major repercussions in terms of health care delivery. For the first time since the introduction of the NHS in 1948, the provision of health and social care services was reliant on a partnership between the government and the private sector. More importantly, however, market forces, rather than the principle of equity, predominated as the guiding factor in meeting health need. This new emphasis on market forces led to an explosion of the private sector in all areas of health and social care, but this was particularly the case in the provision of long-term care facilities, within which women predominated. In fact, because commercial companies were happy to build and expand hospitals and residential care facilities, bed numbers actually increased during this period. Thus, despite the original intention of the government, there was no reduction in health and social care costs (see NAO, 1989).

More importantly, however, though it was clear that factors such as unemployment, poor housing and low income were more damaging to health than lack of health services (see Townsend *et al.*, 1992), the Conservative Government under the leadership of Margaret Thatcher was not committed to changing the situation. Because of her conviction that individuals were responsible for their own health, Thatcher, instead, supported the expansion of media campaigns focusing on health education. Spending on these campaigns rose from £1.6 million in 1979, to £11.4 million in 1988 and reached £30 million in 1995 (Baggott, 1998: 277). Thatcher's government also supported the expansion of cancer-screening programmes, such as that for breast cancer among women. By the mid 1990s, 70 per cent of all women aged 50–64, and 80 per cent of women aged 20–64 were being screened. However, media campaigns and the breast-screening programme have many critics. All the evidence points to the fact that these efforts have made little impact on mortality rates, especially among those on low incomes (for further discussion, see Foster, 1995: 128).

When considered together, the NHS reforms had more critics than supporters at the time of the general election in 1997 (for evaluation of reforms, see Maynard and Bloor, 1996; Klein, 1995; Robinson and Le Grand, 1994). After eighteen years in office, the Conservative Government was replaced by a Labour Government that had among its election promises the reversal of the NHS reforms and the restoration of a comprehensive health care system, based on the original ideology of universal coverage and ease of access. However, it also promised not to increase taxes, thus limiting the amount of money available for public services including health care.

A renewed NHS – empty promises of gender equity?

The Labour Government promised a return to good quality services and to the principles underlying the old NHS – equity, accessibility and comprehensiveness. For the first time in years, health inequalities were highlighted in the new strategy document *Our Healthier Nation* (DoH, 1998a). The principle of equity in the delivery of health and social services was back on the agenda. However, the Labour Government did not intend to return the NHS to its original state nor to abolish the incentives to private provision within the social care sector. In policies described as 'the third way', it soon became obvious that many of the market mechanisms introduced into health and social care services in the 1980s were going to remain – sometimes in another guise.

As the twenty-first century begins, the health service system under a Labour Government is beginning to take shape. To improve quality and maintain standards of care, a *National Institute of Clinical Excellence* and a *Commission for Health Improvement* have been set up. The 'old' health strategy has been revamped, with more emphasis on the need to achieve equality in a range of social and economic factors related to health. The new strategy – *Our Healthier Nation* (DoH, 1998a) – emphasises the need to pay particular attention to areas and groups of people whose health targets are below national averages. This means, for example, that gender-awareness and race-awareness should be built into all health programmes. This is, of course, easier to say than to do.

There are differing views on the impact the new strategy has had on health services in the UK. Women's health movements are already well-established both nationally and internationally (for discussion, see Doyal, 1995) and feminist writers, such as Ann Oakley and Lesley Doyal, are still very critical of the treatment of women within the NHS. Others are more critical of the treatment (or lack of it) of men within the system. As Luck *et al.* (2000: 145) explain:

> Public health policy and programmes lack an adequately gendered perspective i.e. one that takes a balanced view of the health needs of both sexes, rather than present activity which is more focussed and holistic for female health needs but more fragmented for male health needs. The result is that the NHS generally provides health services for males only in indirect and implicit ways.

This is precisely the problem with a health and social care system that does not take gender into account. As long as services are planned simply on the basis of volume of demand, the different needs of men and women are often not met.

One of the major services that should be the most sensitive to the specific needs of each gender is one into which the current government has invested a great deal of hope. This is the primary care service. The plan is that the development of primary care groups (based on current GP practices) will provide access for patients to a wider range of flexible and relevant community services. This, in turn, should shift the balance of care and expenditure from hospital-based services to community-based services. In spite of continual efforts by health administrators since the 1970s to use beds and staff in a more efficient way, the cost of hospital care – and particularly acute care – is still substantial. In 1995–6 the acute sector (including maternity) accounted for 53 per cent of all health care expenditure in England and Wales

(Ham, 1999: 78). As discussed earlier, systematic plans for hospital development have been part of overall health strategies since the 1960s. Changes in medical practice and in medical training have led to a service that now treats more patients in fewer beds. Hospitals now operate with very little spare capacity as day-surgery increases and length of hospital stay decreases. During recent winters, this tightly-run system reached breaking point several times, as emergency admissions spiralled and beds were not available. Efforts by the government to alleviate the situation have included special funding for community services to use beds in the private sector to alleviate this pressure.

What is now clear is that what has become known as 'the partnership' initiative between the public and private sectors will continue to be a characteristic of the health services in the UK, regardless of the government in power. This initiative, begun under Thatcher's Conservative Government of the 1980s, has been continued by the Labour Government. And, while there is no obvious move to privatise publicly-funded and publicly-managed hospitals, there are endless opportunities for joint funding of new hospitals or wards through the Public Finance Initiative (PFI), for the use of private hospital and nursing home beds for publicly-funded patients, and for the use of NHS facilities for private patients (for discussion, see Baggott, 1998: 172–5, 312–13; Ranade, 1994: 46–9). Therefore, there is no real limit on the number of beds that can be made available for health and social care. The commercial sector will respond if financial incentives remain in place, and the non-profit sector will endeavour to fill the gaps in provision for vulnerable groups.

The gender composition of the population in these hospitals and residential facilities remains to be seen. If the trend towards an even larger gap in life expectancy for women and men continues, then the future 'cared-for' population will be predominantly female – that is unless community-based services become a real alternative for people requiring high levels of health and social care.

Summary

- Two of the most important developments in health policy in the early twentieth century were highly gendered in their impact. The first, a public health programme aimed at improving the health of children, highlighted poor mothering as the cause of children's poor health. The second, the introduction of National Health Insurance for employed people, excluded most women and all children from the scheme

- The comprehensive health care system, the NHS, introduced in 1948, led to a rapid expansion in all areas of health service delivery, including a steady increase in the number of beds in hospitals and social care facilities. It also provided the structures and finance for the increasing medicalisation of issues previously outside of its scope. This expansion had more of an impact on women than on men – 'colonising' almost all aspects of childbirth

- Community care policies, initiated in the 1970s, may have led to the discharge from hospital of thousands of people with a mental illness or learning disability, but this, in turn, led to an increasing burden on family carers, most of whom were women

- The NHS reforms, introduced by the Conservative Government under the leadership of Margaret Thatcher, brought with them a new ideology of care – one in which publicly funded hospitals were encouraged to be more market-oriented and commercial providers of health and social care services were welcomed. Efforts to curtail expenditure on hospital care, by reducing bed numbers, were largely unsuccessful because of these two developments, as were media campaigns aimed at reducing health inequalities

- The twenty-first century begins with Tony Blair, leader of the Labour Government, proclaiming the arrival of the 'new' NHS, with its promises of flexibility in service provision and sensitivity to issues of inequalities in health, including gender inequalities. The question remains – are these empty promises?

3 An Empirical Overview

Introduction

As briefly described in Chapter 1, health care provision may be divided into two distinct care categories – primary care and secondary care. Primary care translates into the care provided by the general practitioner (GP), supported by community-based nursing and social services personnel, including social workers and care managers. Secondary care can be summarised as institution-based care and treatment. It includes all care that takes place in hospitals, nursing homes and residential homes for people with a disability or an illness. This chapter provides an empirical overview of health care provision – both physical and mental – in the UK throughout the twentieth century, with an extended discussion on institution-based care (hospitals, nursing homes and social care facilities). Highlighting the importance of gender as a key factor in explaining differences in health care usage, we introduce census data to supplement existing research findings and official statistics. As argued in Chapter 1, the use of census data may be considered particularly appropriate in this instance, as it provides the only comprehensive account of institution-based, or secondary, care in the UK.

Primary care

The term 'primary care' has replaced 'community care' as the new buzzword in health service circles in the UK. As already mentioned, it is care provided by the general practitioner (GP), community nurses and social services personnel. It is hoped that these professionals will work in teams (now called 'Primary Care Groups') to supply basic health and social care services to people in their own homes, with a view to reversing an over-reliance on institution-based care.

The GP service in the UK has always been the province of self-employed practitioners (for a history, see Digby, 1999). Prior to 1911, when National Health Insurance (NHI) was introduced, this was a service available to only a small proportion of the population – those who could afford it from private means or from an employment insurance scheme. The NHI changed this. As we saw in Chapter 2, by the mid 1940s, around half of the population – 21 million people – was covered by NHI and around 90 per cent of GPs were participants in the scheme (Ham, 1999: 8). This injection of funds from the centrally-funded NHI into GP services, prior to the establishment of the National Health Service (NHS) in 1948, was complemented by local authority health services aimed particularly at women and children. Since the 1902 Midwives Act, all midwives had to be certified to practice, but it was not until the 1918 Maternity Act that extra funding was made available to employ health visitors and midwives and to establish infant welfare centres throughout the UK. These services were further expanded in the 1930s to include new ante-natal clinics in many areas. In addition to nurses, welfare officers, who were also employed by the local authority, were part of the primary care service. They replaced Poor Law Officers and were called in only to judge the right of an individual to be admitted freely to a health or welfare institution. These included mental hospitals and publicly funded welfare homes and hospitals that had their origin in Poor Law institutions.

The situation changed radically in 1948, with the introduction of a range of policies, which became collectively known as the Welfare State, including the NHS and a variety of new publicly funded welfare services. GPs remained as self-employed individuals within the NHS, but their services expanded and improved due to an injection of new funds and the increasing professionalisation of all aspects of medical practice. Every member of the population now had a right to free consultations with a GP and to low-cost medicine as prescribed by him (the rate of prescription costs were set by Parliament). The extension of the GP service to the whole population in 1948 was paralleled by an expansion in local authority health and welfare services. In addition to employing health visitors and midwives, these authorities also ran the ambulance service, delivered vaccination and immunisation programmes and developed new welfare services, including an expansion of homes for disabled and older people.

However, the most important developments in primary care services did not happen, according to Ham (1999: 15), until the mid 1960s. These were the expansion of health centres (funded by local authorities) and of community care services. Health centres were funded with a view to encouraging GPs to practise in disadvantaged areas and to work more closely with local authority health and welfare professionals. For example, in 1965, there were 28 health centres in England and Wales, with 215 GPs working in them. By 1989, the number of health centres had increased to 1,320 and the number of GPs working in them to 8,000. This represented 29 per cent of all GPs in Britain at the time (for discussion, see Ham, 1999: 17). By this time, there were also many other GPs working in group practices with no local authority funding. The doctors in these group practices were at the forefront of the development of GP fund-holding practices in the 1990s and of the Primary Care Groups (PCGs) of today. The intention of current government policy is that these PCGs will be led (rather than dominated) by GPs, to improve health and social care services in the community and, thus, to prevent institutionalisation.

It is almost impossible to find statistics that are comparable over time for the primary care service, because of the different management structures under which members of the teams work, and also because of changes in job titles and mode of gathering local authority health and social care data over time. However, there are indications that these services have expanded gradually throughout the twentieth century, and that the 1990s saw a significant increase in their use. Baggott summarises the position succinctly in the following paragraph:

> The pressure on primary care providers intensified considerably in the first half of the 1990s. In England, the number of GP consultations rose by 16 per cent between 1990 and 1994. Over the same period, the number of prescriptions issued increased by 15 per cent. Between 1991/2 and 1994/5 the number of initial contacts by community nurses in England rose by eight per cent (from 2,468,000 to 2,665,000). Health visitors also faced a growing workload, the number of persons visited at home rising from 3,643,000 to 3,711,000 between 1990/1 and 1994/5. (Baggott, 1998: 220)

It is important to note, however, that men and women were not equally served by this significant expansion in primary care services. In other words, not only did more women than men avail themselves of these services, but this was particularly true for consultation with a GP, who is the gatekeeper for all other primary care services. Evidence for the disproportionate use of services among women comes from the General Household Survey of 1992 and 1994. For example, in 1994, 12 per cent of men reported that they had consulted their GP in the previous two-week period, as compared to 17 per cent of women (OPCS, 1996). When attendance is broken down by age, the gender gap seems to be greatest in those aged between 15 and 44 years – young adulthood – the period of greatest health risk for men. For example, in 1992, 9 per cent of men and 18 per cent of women in this age group reported seeing their GP in the previous two weeks (O'Dowd and Jewell, 1998). It is clear from this evidence that, for reasons that will be discussed later, young men are not accessing primary care services, many of which are available only through a GP. In other words, primary care provision seems to be catering adequately for women but not for men, at a time in their lives when they are most in need of health advice.

Secondary care

Secondary care can be summarised as institution-based care and treatment. However, the term 'institution' has such negative connotations that we try to avoid its use unless it seems necessary for the purposes of clarification. As previously explained, secondary care includes all care that takes place in hospitals, nursing homes and residential homes for people with a disability or an illness. In the discussion that follows in this chapter, we include all of the facilities – both physical and mental – designated as health or as social care units in the UK. Later in the book, we will further distinguish between the two sectors – health and social care – in order to make particular points about older people.

The importance of a thorough discussion on secondary care is clear when one realises that it has accounted for the greatest proportion of the NHS budget since its inception in 1948. The costs have been highlighted by health economist, Christopher Ham, who, in analysing NHS expenditure for 1997/8, found that the biggest proportion went on hospital and community health services – 73 per cent – of which 49 per cent was spent on acute hospital care. The total NHS budget for that year was £36,438 million (Ham, 1999: 77–8), reflecting the cost of a consistently significant, albeit fluctuating, population within these health and social care facilities throughout the twentieth century (see Table 3.1).

If we look at the data presented in Table 3.1, we see that the size of the population in health and social care facilities increased substantially between 1921 and 1971 – from 491,208 to 654,723 – an increase of 163,515 people. The trend changed dramatically during the 1970s when the total population decreased substantially. As a result, by 1981 the population occupying health and social care beds was 428,994 people, the lowest level recorded in the twentieth century. This was a direct result of a change in medical practice – the move to day-surgery within physical health care and to day-treatment within mental health care. Although, as discussed in Chapter 2, this move was facilitated by policy-makers concerned with reducing health expenditure, it was made possible by technological advances in medical practice.

Table 3.1 The population in health and social care facilities in the UK, 1921–91

Census year	Number of occupants
1921/26	491,208
1931/37	591,721
1951	603,854
1961	647,033
1971	654,723
1981	428,994
1991	562,544

Note: In addition to hospitals and residential facilities for disabled and older people, children's homes are included for the census periods prior to 1951 in Britain and prior to 1971 in Northern Ireland. The notable decline in occupancy levels between 1971 and 1981 may be explained by the large number of individuals ($n = 229,990$) who were classified as non-residents in these facilities in Britain in 1981.

Source: England & Wales and Scotland Census, 1921, 1931, 1951, 1961, 1971, 1981, 1991; Northern Ireland Census, 1926, 1937, 1951, 1961, 1971, 1981, 1991.

While it is clear in the statistics for 1981 that the steady growth in the population resident in health and social care facilities was halted during the 1970s, this was not the beginning of a new downward trend. In 1991, the population in residential health and social care facilities increased again by 133,550 to 562,544 people. Furthermore, a closer look at the statistics for 1981 reveals that it is unlikely that the level of actual bed provision had been reduced during this period, as there were 229,990 people classified as non-resident patients in that year. This means that in spite of the apparent downturn in bed occupancy, it is likely that both bed numbers and people using these beds increased during the 1970s and early 1980s. In the last decade of the century, the emphasis on cost-cutting within the overall health budget (Ham, 1999: 28–35) and the highly publicised cuts in hospital beds will, no doubt, have reduced bed numbers and had an impact on the

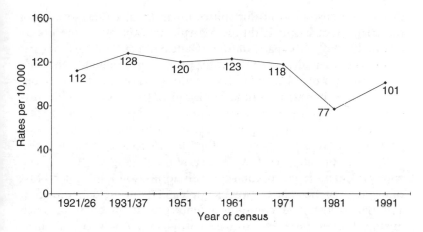

Figure 3.1 Rates per 10,000 of the population in health and social care facilities in the UK, 1921–91

Source: England & Wales and Scotland Census, 1921, 1931, 1951, 1961, 1981, 1991; Northern Ireland Census, 1926, 1937, 1951, 1971, 1981, 1991.

volume of people using these beds on a daily basis. However, this will not be clear until after the publication of statistics from the 2001 census.

Another way of looking at these statistics is in terms of the total general UK population. In other words, what do these statistics say about levels of institutionalisation in the society as a whole? The simplest way to answer this question is to use the same numbers to calculate how many people were in health and social care facilities per 10,000 of the total population in the UK. Figure 3.1 provides this information.

This figure 3.1 gives us a slightly different picture than that shown in Table 3.1. While 1981 still remains the year in which the lowest level of institutionalisation is recorded (only 77 people per 10,000 of the population), the downward trend had begun in the 1960s. However, the main trends are clear. The level of institutionalisation in health and social care facilities rose during the 1920s, remained pretty stable during the 1930s, 1940s and 1950s, reduced during the 1960s and 1970s, but began to increase again during the 1980s and early 1990s.

What is particularly interesting about this increase is the fact that it demonstrates the difficulties inherent in trying to control the quantity of hospital and residential care available to the population. In the early part of the twentieth century, health care, particularly that delivered in institutions – hospitals for the sick and homes for disabled and older people – was offered by a mixture of providers. It was, according to Baggott (1998: 86) a 'rather disorganised and complex mixture of private and public services'. The main provider within the public sector was local government, supported by a modicum of central funding. In contrast, the providers within the private sector were diverse, consisting of commercial enterprises and large voluntary organisations, some of which continue in existence today (for example, The Nuffield Foundation and Barnardos). The commercial enterprises ranged from small nursing homes, owned and managed by one person to large hospitals owned and managed by companies. The best examples of individually-run private establishments were the private madhouses of the nineteenth century, some of which survived into the early twentieth century (Parry-Jones, 1972). In spite of the diversity of provision, the quality of care was considered extremely inadequate but, as we can see from the information in Table 3.1 and Figure 3.1, the level of total provision continued to increase during the 1920s and 1930s. This happened in spite of the funding difficulties experienced by voluntary hospitals and local authorities alike, and the personal financial difficulties experienced by the population at large (for discussion, see Abel-Smith, 1994; Prior, 1993). After 1948, when the NHS was established and the management of these diverse institutions transferred to a central body, the upward trend continued, in spite of efforts by politicians and health administrators to keep costs down.

It was not until the early 1980s that a downturn in the level of institutionalisation in relation to the general population as well as in the actual number of people in residential health and social care facilities began to show. The reaction to this trend was mostly positive. The anti-institution movement, spurred on by the writings of Goffman (1961), Laing (1960) and Barton (1959), welcomed it because it showed a commitment to reducing numbers of people using this form of treatment. Politicians and health administrators welcomed it because it meant a reduction in costs. However, doctors and other health professionals found that their workload had not lightened, mainly due to the fact that patient numbers continued to increase, despite a reduction in the number of available beds.

The downward trend did not last long and, by the early 1990s, the numbers of people in health and social care beds had begun to climb again. This parallelled policy changes in health and social care, which encouraged private providers to enter the market. In an effort to bring new funding into health care, the NHS reforms, introduced by the Thatcher Government during the 1980s, resulted in the expansion of private hospitals concentrating on surgical interventions and of private nursing and social care homes concentrating on the care of an ageing population (for discussion, see Le Grand and Bartlett, 1993; Wistow *et al.*, 1994).

Mind or body?

As previously explained, institution-based care may be divided into two main areas: treatment for physical illness and disability – often referred to as 'general' health care – and treatment for mental illness – usually referred to as 'mental' health care. We will now disaggregate the population receiving institution-based care, in order to estimate the level of secondary care provision for physical and mental health separately (Figure 3.2).

Figure 3.2 shows a very simple trend. The population in mental health facilities formed less than one-third of the total population in health and social care facilities for most of the twentieth century, dropping steeply to under 10 per cent during the 1980s. As might be expected, from what we know of the changing attitudes to hospital-based mental health care – from positive to negative – the proportion of the population in mental health beds began to decrease during the second half of the twentieth century. Although Figure 3.2 does not include data for 1961 (because of the absence of data for Northern Ireland), the 1961 census in England and Wales shows that the proportion of the population in mental health beds (in relation to the total cared-for population) had already begun to decrease (Prior and Hayes, 2001b: 405). This is interesting, as it supports the theory that the 'drug revolution' in psychiatric treatment of the 1950s had already made an impact on mental hospital populations before community care policies were introduced (see Jones, 1993). What is even

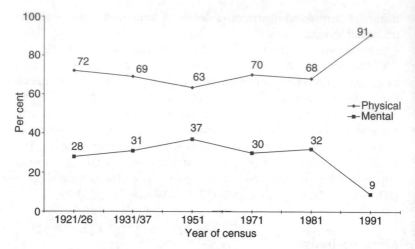

Figure 3.2 Differences in levels of bed occupancy in physical and mental health and social care facilities in the UK, 1921–91

Source: England & Wales and Scotland Census, 1921, 1931, 1951, 1971, 1981, 1991; Northern Ireland Census, 1926, 1937, 1951, 1971, 1981, 1991.

more interesting, however, is that this decrease in the mental hospital population did not result in an overall decline within the institution-based population as a whole. Rather, as the data in Table 3.1 and Figure 3.2 clearly show, the reduction in the population in mental health facilities from the 1950s onwards was accompanied by a parallel increase in the population in general health care facilities – a pattern that continues to this day. As the last decade of the twentieth century began, almost 91 per cent of the population in health and social care facilities were receiving care for a physical illness or disability as compared to 9 per cent for mental illness.

On the question of gender

As with other areas of health care provision, secondary care impacts differently on men and women in the UK and has done so consistently throughout the twentieth century. Because we are concerned here with a simple overview of the situation, we will merely highlight the most outstanding gender differences in the

Table 3.2 Gender differences in levels of bed occupancy in physical and mental health and social care facilities in the UK, 1921–91

Year	Physical (%)	Mental (%)	Number of occupants
Panel A: Men			
1921/26	75.2	24.8	254,818
1931/37	72.5	27.5	305,292
1951	62.2	37.8	270,722
1961	—	—	270,248
1971	62.5	37.5	253,125
1981	53.6	46.4	142,192
1991	84.7	15.3	171,493
Panel B: Women			
1921/26	67.7	32.3	236,390
1931/37	65.9	34.1	286,429
1951	63.7	36.3	333,132
1961	—		376,785
1971	74.0	26.0	401,598
1981	75.7	24.3	286,802
1991	93.3	6.7	391,051

Note: Because of the absence of distinguishing data for Northern Ireland, a separate UK figure for physical and mental health and social care facilities could not be calculated for the 1961 census period. The notable decline in occupancy levels between 1971 and 1981 may be explained by the large number of males ($n = 86,091$) and females ($n = 143,899$) who were classified as non-residents in these facilities in Britain in 1981.

Source: England & Wales and Scotland Census, 1921, 1931, 1951, 1971, 1981, 1991; Northern Ireland Census, 1926, 1937, 1951, 1971, 1981, 1991.

use of secondary care facilities to emerge from census data, differentiating between physical and mental health care. These data are shown in Table 3.2. Panel A presents the results for men and Panel B shows the equivalent data for women.

Table 3.2 shows two quite different patterns of changing health service use by men and women. The first is that, while the male population in health and social care facilities was larger than the equivalent female population in the 1920s – 254,818 males and

236,390 females, the situation had reversed by the last decade of the twentieth century. In 1991, the female population in these facilities far outstripped the male population – 391,051 females and 171,493 males. In other words, contrary to popular opinion, women have not always been the higher users of secondary care. The second compelling fact to emerge is that in 1981, when bed occupancy for both men and women dropped sharply, the gender patterns were quite different for physical and mental health care. In that year, the male population was almost equally divided between physical and mental health facilities, while the majority of females (76 per cent) were in physical care facilities. What this means in terms of the de-institutionalisation policies is that the efforts to discharge men from mental hospitals during the 1970s were not as successful as might have been expected. The final important fact to emerge from this brief analysis of census data is that, by the last decade of the twentieth century, the female population in institution-based care was almost completely concentrated in the physical care sector (93 per cent), while the imbalance was not so pronounced in the male population. The reasons for these very different patterns of service use among women and men form the basis for the discussion that follows in the remainder of the book.

Summary

- Women are much higher users of the continually expanding primary care service
- The population in residential health and social care facilities is on the increase again, after a brief downturn during the 1970s
- Women now form the vast majority of this population, though men were in the majority in the early decades of the twentieth century
- Although the vast majority of men and women are now concentrated in the physical care sector or facilities catering for physical illness and disability, this is particularly the case among women

Part II
Stereotypes Fullfilled?

4 Gender and Physical Health

Introduction

The academic debate on gender and physical health, which began in the 1970s (Mechanic, 1978; Nathanson, 1977; Waldron, 1976), has continued since then on both sides of the Atlantic. For most of this time, it has been generally accepted that women experience more illness than men and are higher users of health services but that, in spite of this, they live longer. As briefly discussed in Chapter 1, these facts are summarised in the phrase – 'women are sicker but men die quicker'. This seemingly contradictory statement is based on substantial research evidence of higher levels of morbidity in the female population and higher levels of mortality in the male population.

Some researchers, however, have questioned the taken-for-granted assumptions underlying this argument and the generalisations that inevitably flow from it (see Arber and Cooper, 1999;

47

Macintyre *et al.*, 1996). While not disagreeing with the basic tenet – health is gendered because all opportunities, including life chances, are greatly influenced by gender – these writers point to the need to take into account the impact of changing gender roles on health. They also suggest a more rigorous analysis of differences within the male and female sub-populations in relation to age, ethnicity, geographic location and type of illness. It is with these recommendations in mind that this chapter focuses not only on gender differences in mortality and morbidity rates in physical health within the UK but also on the gendered, albeit changing, nature of health service use within the secondary care sector.

Mortality rates – men die quicker?

Death rates are higher for men than women in the UK for most disease categories and in every age group (see Baggott, 1998: 23; DoH, 1996). This pattern is reflected in overall mortality rates, which have been consistently higher for men than for women throughout the twentieth century. At the beginning of the century, a new-born male could expect to live for 46 years and a new-born female for 49 years. By the end of the century, the life expectancy for both genders had increased, as had the difference between the two. A new-born male can now expect to live to around 75 years and a new-born female to around 80 years of age (see Ham, 1999: 185–8; Baggott, 1998: 3).

Box 4.1 Gender and life expectancy in the UK

- Most of the girls born in the UK in 2002 will still be alive in 2082
- Most of the boys born in the UK in 2002 will not be alive after 2077

The overall improvement in health was due mainly to public health interventions at the beginning of the century, most notably universal sanitation schemes and the control of infectious diseases.

However, as diseases such as cholera, typhoid, tuberculosis and measles disappeared, others have replaced them. These include cancers, heart disease and AIDS. Currently, 'the four main causes of death in men are diseases of circulation, cancer, accidents and suicide' (O'Dowd and Jewell, 1998: 1). By far the commonest causes of death are diseases of the circulatory system, but those caused by accidents and suicides are substantial enough to give rise to great concern.

The following data from the office of the Chief Medical Officer for England and Wales for 1995 give a picture of the major diseases specifically affecting men. As one would expect, the main causes of death vary greatly by age. In 1995, ischaemic heart disease and cerebro-vascular disease (stroke) together accounted for 29 per cent of deaths in men aged 35–54 years and 37 per cent of those aged 55–74 years. Lung cancer, which increased consistently as a cause of death for men in the first half of the century, has now begun to decrease steadily. However, it still accounted for 8 per cent of deaths in men aged 35–54 years and 11 per cent in those aged 55–74 years in 1995. For younger men the causes of death were quite different – 22 per cent were caused by suicide and undetermined injury and 16 per cent by car accidents in those aged 15–34 years (for these and other data, see DoH, 1996). The incidence of suicide, in particular among young men, has given rise to great concern in recent years and has been linked to a possible increase in mental health problems in this group (see Chapter 9).

This picture of male health and illness in the UK is echoed in the USA. There, the average life-span for men is now seven years less than that for women and mortality rates in the fifteen leading causes of death are higher for men than for women. According to Courtenay (2000: 1385):

> Men's age-adjusted death rate for heart disease, for example, is two times higher than women's, and men's cancer death rate is 1.5 times higher . . . Nearly three out of four persons who die from heart attacks before age 65 are men.

This is not to deny, however, the importance of these diseases in predicting mortality rates among women. For example, despite the introduction of a range of public health initiatives, such as the expansion of cancer-screening programmes in the 1990s, cancer

– particularly breast cancer and cancers of the genito-urinary system – also remains one of the major causes of death in women. As Baggott (1998: 23) explains:

> Breast cancer and cancers of the genito-urinary system are major causes of death in women. Every year, around 15,000 women in the UK die from breast cancer, the biggest cause of death from cancer among women. A further 2,000 women in the UK die from cervical cancer.

Other serious illnesses, such as lung cancer and heart disease, though manifesting much lower mortality rates than for men, also result in the death of a substantial number of women (Baggott, 1998: 7; DoH, 1998a: Fig. 12). Furthermore, statistics for both of these diseases are changing. In relation to lung cancer, for example, mortality rates for women have been increasing, lowering the differential between men and women. However, as Waldron (2000) has shown in relation to trends in the USA, mortality rates from lung cancer are highly related to cigarette-smoking behaviour (with a time lag of 20–30 years) and vary greatly by age and country studied. Using a sex mortality ratio (male to female) to indicate trends, Waldron (2000: 156) summarises the situation in the USA from 1950 to 1990 as follows:

> During the early part of this period, lung cancer mortality increased more rapidly for males, so sex mortality ratios increased. Conversely, during the later part of the period, lung cancer mortality increased more rapidly for females, so sex mortality ratios decreased. Thus sex mortality ratios for lung cancer increased from 4.6 in 1950 to a maximum of 6.7 in 1960, and then decreased to 2.3 in 1990.

Trends for mortality from lung cancer in the UK are similar to those in the USA, so it is likely that current smoking behaviour among women will determine the level of mortality from lung cancer in twenty years time. The indications are that women are less likely than men to be current smokers and that their average consumption of cigarettes is lower, but the gap is not very wide. For example, in 1994, British men were found to be more likely than women to smoke – with 28 per cent of men and 26 per cent of women defining themselves as current smokers. In addition, men smoked more cigarettes per week – with an average of 114 cigarettes – than did women – with an average of 97 ciga-

rettes per week (Bunting 1997: 215). However, these differences
may disappear in the future as there is some evidence that men
are reducing their cigarette consumption and women are increasing theirs (DoH, 1996).

Even in relation to heart disease (referred to either as coronary or ischaemic heart disease), although women continue to
have much lower mortality rates than men, rates for both have
declined over the past fifty years (Charlton and Murphy, 1997a:
150–2). Furthermore, it still remains a major cause of death in
older women throughout the western world. For example, in the
USA, coronary heart disease is now 'the single most important
cause of death in post-menopausal women, killing half a million
a year' (Doyal, 1995: 17). We do not have an equivalent figure for
the UK, but mortality estimates for all diseases of the circulatory
system in England and Wales suggest the absence of a gender gap
in relation to this area of ill health. For example, in 1994, whereas
diseases of the circulatory system accounted for 44 per cent of
female deaths in Britain, the equivalent figure among males was,
in fact, 1 per cent lower at 43 per cent. Ischaemic heart disease
remains the most important of this group of diseases, accounting
for 57 per cent of these deaths in that year (Charlton and Murphy,
1997a: 44). As in the USA, the age at which these deaths occur
is generally older among women than among men. There are
some indications to suggest, however, that the increased risk of
death from heart disease for middle-aged women that emerged
in mortality statistics for the 1970s, decreased again during the
1980s (Charlton and Murphy, 1997a: 152).

Another important mortality statistic related to both gender
and age is that arising from accidents and violence. In the late
1980s, in the under-35-year-old population, 35 per cent of female
deaths in the UK, as opposed to 70 per cent of male deaths, were
caused by accidents and violence (Doyal, 1995: 20). In other
words, it could be said that young women were much less prone
than young men to death from violence or from accidents – at
home, at work or on the road. However, the picture is not as
clear now, though, overall, women are still less likely to die from
accidents and violence than are men. In the context of an overall
decrease in accident-related deaths in both the UK and the USA,
it appears that gender differentials have decreased in relation to
car accidents and accidents at work. This is due to the increasing number of women driving cars and engaging in blue-collar

employment, making them more likely to have accidents in both situations. Among older people, women show higher level of mortality due to accidents (usually in the home) than do men (Charlton and Murphy, 1997a: Fig. 4.16, p. 52). This is probably due to the fact that women live longer than men rather than to any other cause.

In summary, then, although women continue to experience much lower mortality rates than men across a variety of illnesses, the old adage that 'men die quicker' is not as clear-cut as it seems. Our arguments in support of this proposition are threefold. First, as our review of the evidence clearly suggests, while mortality rates are much higher among men than women in relation to certain illness, such as lung disease and heart disease, this is by no means a universal finding. Second, even among long-standing differential mortality rates, such as deaths arising from accidents, there is some evidence to suggest that the gender gap is narrowing over time. Finally, these statistics demonstrate the importance of distinguishing not only causes of death and types of illness when considering gender differences in mortality rates but also the important mediating effects of age or stage in the life-cycle.

Morbidity rates – women are sicker?

As previously explained, morbidity rates are based either on self-reported health status (as recorded by a researcher) or on a medical diagnosis made during a visit to a health professional (usually a doctor). Most of the research on populations in the USA and the UK suggests that in each of these situations men are less forthcoming than women about their health problems. Verbrugge (1989) found, for example, in a study of white adults in Detroit, that men had lower morbidity rates and lower levels of health care use than women in 60 out of 67 different measures of health status. This finding was backed up by later studies which showed that, even among men and women with similar health problems, 'men are significantly more likely than women to have had no recent physician contact' (Courtenay, 2000: 1386). This pattern of lower health service use by men than by women has now been generally accepted within the research community, as has the fact that men report better health than women.

In the UK, the evidence for the lower reporting of illness by men is found mainly through the General Household Survey (GHS) carried out annually by the Office for National Statistics (ONS). This is supplemented by data from the 1984 Health and Lifestyle Survey (HALS) and the 1993 Health Survey for England (HSFE). For example, in the GHS, men have traditionally reported lower rates of long-standing illness and lower levels of health service use than women (OPCS, 1996, 1994). In the 1994 GHS, a slightly smaller proportion of men reported that they had attended an out-patient clinic in the previous three months than had women – 14 per cent for men as compared to 15 per cent for women. They also reported a much lower level of attendance at their general practitioner (GP) in the previous two weeks – 12 per cent for men and 17 per cent for women (OPCS, 1996). By the 1996 GHS, the gender gap in GP attendance had widened slightly – with 13 per cent of men and 19 per cent of women reporting they had seen their GP in the two weeks before the survey (ONS, 1998).

However, this gender differential in reporting of illness cannot be taken as given across all age groups. For example, when Macintyre and her colleagues at the Medical Research Council research unit at Glasgow examined the GHS data for 1992 more closely, they found that the female excess in reporting long-standing illness was present only in the over-75-year-old population (Macintyre *et al.*, 1996):

> in 1992, males were reported as having more long-standing illness in early childhood, and that thereafter up to the age of 74 there was little difference in reported prevalence between males and females; it was only after 75 that there was a female excess of more than one per cent. (Macintyre *et al.*, 1996: 618)

There were similar findings in the 1994 GHS, with an identical proportion of both men and women aged under 65 years – 32 per cent – reporting having a long-standing illness. Among those aged 65 years or older, men again reported lower rates then women (OPCS, 1996). Perhaps, the pattern is changing, with younger men more likely to report illness than previous generations. However, the empirical evidence is not yet sufficient enough to support this claim. For the moment, it seems that admitting to illness – whether to a doctor or to a researcher – is still seen as a sign of male weakness (for further discussion, see Luck *et al.*, 2000). In other words, while there is some debate as to whether the first part of the old adage – 'men die quicker' – is still correct, the second part – 'women are sicker' – still appears to hold true, especially in relation to the reporting of illness.

Sociological perspectives on gender differences in health

What may explain these differences in mortality and morbidity rates among men and women? As outlined in Chapter 1, four general causal explanations – biomedical, psychosocial, epidemiological and socio-political – have been put forward to account for gender differences in health (Kawachi *et al.*, 1999: 89). As one would expect, sociological accounts of this phenomenon have tended to discount the biomedical explanation in favour of derivative explanations from the latter three. To date, three sociological explanations have been put forward to explain gender differences in physical health patterns. These are lifestyle (derivative of the psychosocial explanation), under-reporting of illness (derivative of the epidemiological explanation) and socioeconomic inequalities (derivative of the socio-political approach). It is important to note, however, that, while two of these explanations – life-style and under-reporting of illness – specifically focus on gender differences in mortality and morbidity statistics, the third – socio-economic inequalities – discounts gender as a primary factor in explaining differences in ill-health. Rather, according to this explanation, it is class, and not gender, that accounts for differences in health inequalities not only between men and women but also within both the male and female sub-populations as a whole.

Box 4.2 Sociological explanations for gender differences in health patterns

- Life-style
- Under-reporting of illness
- Socio-economic inequalities

Focusing initially on the first explanation, or differences in life-style, many of the major causes of death in men (cardiovascular diseases, lung cancer and car accidents) have been linked to life-style. This is particularly the case in the public health literature. According to this perspective, it is over-use of alcohol or ciga-rettes, lack of physical exercise, poor diet and exposure to ex-cessive stress, that not only leads to ill-health, but specifically predisposes individuals, the majority of whom are men, to cardiovascular problems and lung cancer (see Jacobson *et al.*, 1991). As previously explained, these arguments are consistent with research in the UK. For example, not only are men more likely than women to smoke, but males have much higher rates of alcohol consumption than females. In the GHS for 1995, men admitted to a weekly average alcohol consumption of 15.4 units and women to 5.4 units (ONS, 1997: Table 15.14). Men are also significantly more likely to die as a result of vio-lence or from accident-related incidences than women (Doyal, 1995: 20).

Similar arguments are evident in the public health literature in the USA. Policy statements from the office of the US Surgeon General in the mid-1990s suggest that half of all deaths could be prevented through life-style changes. This suggestion has been supported by numerous health studies from a range of researchers, particularly in relation to the male sub-population (for discussion, see Woolf *et al.*, 1996). Health monitoring systems on nationally representative samples in the USA have found that men, particu-larly young men, engage much more often in behaviours detri-mental to health than do women. As Courtenay (2000: 1386) explains:

> Data from one such system indicate that the prevalence of risk behaviours among adults is more common among men than women for all but three of fourteen (non sex-specific) behav-iours, including smoking, drinking and driving, using safety belts, getting health screenings, and awareness of medical conditions.

In other words, according to this perspective, it is this factor – the greater tendency among men to engage in behaviour that puts their health at risk – that explains gender differences in health. The 'life-style' argument has been used widely in recent years to 'blame' people for their own poor health. As explained earlier, one consequence of this was a tendency in UK health policies under the Conservative governments of the 1980s and early 1990s to emphasise individual rather than community responsibility for health, as reflected in the growth of media campaigns on health education during the Thatcher era.

The life-style argument – or gender differences in risk-taking behaviour – is not the only explanation advanced to explain inequalities in health. An alternative perspective, which specifically focuses on differences in morbidity patterns, suggests that it is the under-reporting of illness among males that provides the best explanation. As with the life-style argument, empirical evidence in support of this position is available in both the UK and the USA. For example, as previously explained, not only are men significantly more likely than women to have had no recent physician contact, but they are also less likely to say that they experience any illness (see Courtenay, 2000; OPCS, 1996, 1994). In other words, it is this factor – the lower health service use and reporting of illness among men than women – that explains gender differences in morbidity rates.

It is important to note, however, that the gender difference in the reporting of illness is not consistent across all age groups. In fact, when long-standing illnesses are considered, female excess in reporting illness is confined to populations over 75 years of age (Macintyre et al., 1996). This is not to deny, however, significant differences in morbidity rates among men and women. Irrespective of whether the UK or the USA is considered, as a group, men report lower levels of illness and demonstrate lower levels of health care use than women. Thus, as previously explained, for the moment at least, it seems that admitting to illness – whether to a doctor or to a researcher – is seen as an almost exclusively female characteristic.

We turn now to our final sociological explanation – socio-economic inequalities. According to this perspective, it is class, and not gender, that accounts for differences in health inequalities not only between men and women but also within both the male and female sub-populations as a whole. In other words, supporters of this approach suggest that the primary factor in explaining health inequalities is variation in socio-economic position and this relationship remains irrespective of whether differences in gender, ethnicity or even geographical area are included in the analysis.

Empirical evidence in support of this position is available for both the UK and the USA.

Life expectancy, incidence of lung cancer and death due to accidents, for example, have been consistently shown to vary enormously by class (DoH, 1998a; Wilkinson, 1996; Power, 1994). Life expectancy decreases and incidence of illness increases as socio-economic position decreases. For example, men in the lower income groups have much higher levels of mortality and of morbidity than those in higher income groups. More specifically, a man born into social class I (professional) has an extra seven years life expectancy than a man born into classes IV or V (partly skilled and unskilled). In addition, this class differential among males is reflected in self-reported long-standing illnesses and in every aspect of health measured in the Health and Lifestyle Survey (see OPCS, 1996; Harding, 1995; Blaxter, 1990).

Of course, socio-economic inequalities in health are not confined to the male population. While the overall average life-span for women in the UK is approximately 80 years, 5–6 years longer than for men, this varies enormously by socio-economic grouping and ethnic background. For example, women married to professional men have a much longer life expectancy than women married to semi-skilled or unskilled men, due to widening class differences in the risk of dying from lung cancer, heart disease and breast cancer (Drever and Whitehead, 1997; OPCS, 1996).

In addition to class inequalities in health, those in relation to ethnicity are receiving more attention. It is generally accepted that women from the white population have a longer life expectancy than have those from ethnic minorities, although the reasons for this have not yet been fully explored. For example, research by Balarajan (1991), in the Asian community in England and Wales, found that the mortality rate for coronary health disease for people born in the 'Indian sub-continent is 36 per cent higher for men and 46 per cent higher for women when compared with the national average'. There is also some evidence that there is a higher incidence of renal disease and of a specific musculoskeletal disease known as SLE among specific ethnic groups in the UK (Charlton and Murphy, 1997b: 121, 148). It is important to note, however, that these specific diseases are unlikely to be the main cause of poor health and high rates of mortality among women or men. Rather, it is much more likely that health inequalities within both the female and male population has much more to do with economic differentials. Thus, although women may have a health advantage on men because of their gender, according to this perspective, this advantage often disappears in the context of other socio-economic factors such as low income and ethnic background.

Secondary care services – women replace men

As we have seen earlier, it can be said that, in general, women admit to higher levels of physical illness and make greater use of primary health care services than do men (for discussion, see Macintyre *et al.*, 1996). In the UK, the GP is the gatekeeper to all specialist services, including outpatient consultations at a specialist clinic, and admissions for care or treatment in a hospital or social care facility. This is not to suggest, however, that this is the only channel for admission to hospital or residential care facility. For example, in 1999 and 2000, emergency admissions accounted for around one-third of all hospital admissions in England and Wales (DoH, 2000). In both years, however, they constituted a minority of patients with the bulk of admissions entering via the GP referral route. As men are lower users of GP services than are women, as shown in the GHS, we would expect, therefore, that they are also likely to be lower users of secondary care services, such as hospitals, nursing homes and residential social care facilities.

Is this, in fact, the case? Are women higher users of these services than men? In other words, do their higher levels of reported illness also translate into their greater use of secondary care services for physical illness and disability? The data presented in Chapter 3 provided some indirect evidence in support of this proposition. Based on a comparison of the populations in physical and mental health care facilities, the results suggested that although the vast majority of men and women in institutional care are now concentrated in physical care facilities, this is particularly the case among women. To what extent, however, does this finding also remain when a more direct and comprehensive examination of this issue is undertaken? In other words, when men and women are directly compared, are women higher users of secondary care (physical illness and disability) than men? Table

Table 4.1 Gender differences in levels of bed occupancy in physical health and social care facilities in the UK, 1921–91

Year	Men (%)	Women (%)	Number of occupants
1921/26	54.5	45.5	351,364
1931/37	54.0	46.0	410,089
1951	44.2	55.8	380,604
1971	34.7	65.3	455,664
1981	26.0	74.0	293,303
1991	28.5	71.5	510,165

Note: Because of the absence of distinguishing data between physical and mental health facilities in Northern Ireland, a UK figure could not be calculated for the 1961 census period.

Source: England & Wales and Scotland Census, 1921, 1931, 1951, 1971, 1981, 1991; Northern Ireland Census, 1926, 1937, 1951, 1971, 1981, 1991.

4.1 provides the answer to this question by calculating the proportion of men and women in physical health care facilities, usually referred to as the 'general' health care sector. Mental health care will be discussed separately in Chapter 8. As with earlier discussions of secondary care services, this information is derived from an analysis of census data on occupants of all health and social care beds in the UK in all but one decade – 1961 – since the 1920s. This year was omitted as a figure for the UK could not be calculated, due to the absence of data distinguishing between physical and mental health facilities in Northern Ireland.

The data is Table 4.1 confirm our expectation that women are higher users of these services than men. For the second half of the twentieth century, women were in the majority in the population in residential health and social care facilities in the UK. The trend seems set to continue, as the proportion of women in these facilities continued to rise in 1981, in spite of a downturn in the number of occupied beds – from 455,664 in 1971 to 293,303 in 1981 – a decade earlier. It is interesting to note, however, that the higher use of these facilities by women seemed to have begun just around the time of the establishment of the NHS in 1948. Before that, men were slightly higher users of these services than women.

The reason for the increasing proportion of women in these facilities from the late 1940s onwards is hard to fathom. Either it reflects a higher level of illness in the male as compared to the female population in the early decades of the century or it reflects a higher level of reporting of illness by men. As the latter is unlikely, we will have to assume a higher level of illness among men than among women, possibly related to working in dangerous environments. During the Second World War, it is likely that part of the trend reversal was due to the immersion of the male population in the war effort (for discussion of the impact of war on health service use, see Abel-Smith, 1964; Aubrey, 1941). However, it is unlikely that war was the most significant factor in this case, as the new gender pattern of women predominating continued throughout the second half of the twentieth century, increasing steadily as time went on.

By 1981, women outnumbered men in residential health and social care facilities by almost three to one. This was in spite of a reduction in the population classified as resident in these facilities in that year, due to a change in treatment and care regimes, which channelled patients into day-surgery and day-care (for statistics, see Chapter 3; for further discussion, see Ranade, 1994: 152). We have no reason to believe that the option of day-surgery or other day-treatments was not offered on an equal basis to men and women. However, as the statistics for 1971 and 1981 show, this change in medical practice served to increase further the gender gap in the use of residential health and social care services in the UK. In 1981, the imbalance between men and women was greatest, with women occupying 74 per cent and men occupying only 26 per cent of all health and social care beds – a gender gap of 48 per cent. Ten years later, although the provision of day-treatment and day-care continued to increase, the size of the resident (overnight) population in health and social care facilities rose dramatically to its highest point during the twentieth century – 510,165 people. The population in these facilities continued to be overwhelmingly female – with women occupying 71.5 per cent and men occupying 28.5 per cent of these beds. As will be shown in Chapter 6, most of this expansion took place in the social care sector (residential care homes) rather than in the health care sector (hospitals and nursing homes), but, regardless of the sector, women dominated in this 'cared for' population.

Gender differences in health service use – the importance of region

Within the UK, there is great geographical variation in the health of the population. This variation is highlighted in the literature on inequalities in health. For example, northern areas report worse health than southern areas (Townsend *et al.*, 1992) and Scotland and Northern Ireland report higher morbidity and mortality rates than England and Wales (Ham, 1999: 191; Baggott, 1998: 15; Carstairs and Morris, 1991). The higher level of illness in the populations of Scotland and Northern Ireland was confirmed in the census. Both Scotland and Northern Ireland had a higher level of use of secondary care services than England and Wales for most of the twentieth century.

In the 1990s, Northern Ireland showed the greatest difference from the average, with a much higher rate of bed occupancy, in terms of the general population, than either Scotland or England and Wales. In 1991, Northern Ireland had 139 occupied beds per 10,000 of the general population, Scotland 106, and England and Wales 99. These statistics in themselves are startling because they reveal that Northern Ireland has, by far, the highest level of bed occupancy within the UK. What this means in terms of the health status of the population, however, is open to debate. The high level of health service use can be seen, on the one hand, to indicate worse levels of health in the Northern Ireland population. However, it could also be used to show excessive provision of secondary care services. Both arguments have been put forward in the past, with more supporters for the former than the latter (see SSI (NI), 1998).

To what extent, do these regional differences in secondary care provision in the early 1990s also result in a differing gender balance across their respective 'cared for' populations? As the data in Table 4.2 show, while women predominated in these facilities in all parts of the UK in 1991, Northern Ireland is, once again, the outlier, with Scotland showing similar gender patterns to England and Wales.

If we look at the data in Table 4.2, one gender pattern is consistent throughout the UK – women are much higher users of health and social care facilities than men. In fact, the gender balance and, consequently, the gender gap was almost identical in Scotland

Table 4.2 Gender differences in levels of bed occupancy in physical health and social care facilities in the UK by region, 1991

Region	Men (%)	Women (%)	Gender gap (%)	Number of occupants
England & Wales	28.2	71.8	−44	449,114
Scotland	28.4	71.6	−43	42,407
Northern Ireland	35.2	64.8	−30	18,644

Source: England & Wales, Scotland, and Northern Ireland Census, 1991.

to that in England and Wales, with women constituting 72 per cent of the population in these facilities. It can be concluded from this that, although research in the past has shown that on a number of health indicators Scotland is different from England and Wales, this is not the case in this particular instance. However, this may not contradict other findings on higher rates and different patterns of illness in Scotland. As will be discussed in Chapter 6, the population in residential health and social care facilities is dominated numerically by older people (aged 65 years and over) and is based primarily in the social care sector. Although the gender trends in the use of these services are similar in Scotland to those in England and Wales, this may be due to a convergence in demographic trends rather than any change in specific disease patterns.

Northern Ireland, however, has quite a different pattern in the population using residential health and social care services. In 1991, although the general pattern of women predominating was similar, the proportion of men was much higher than in Scotland or England and Wales − 35 per cent in Northern Ireland as compared with 28 per cent elsewhere. This also meant that the gender gap for Northern Ireland was much smaller than elsewhere − at 30 per cent as compared with 44 per cent in England and Wales and 43 per cent in Scotland. As mentioned earlier, Northern Ireland also had a much higher rate of bed occupancy when considered in terms of the general population. This means that it has by far the highest rate of bed occupancy for men than any other area of the UK. In other words, the men in Northern Ireland appear to be less healthy than their counterparts in Scotland or

England and Wales. This would fit with other health statistics on Northern Ireland, which show higher levels of disadvantage and higher levels of illness and disability than in other parts of the UK [SSI (NI), 1998]. However, the findings do not contradict the consistent pattern of higher usage of residential health and social care services (hospitals, nursing homes and care homes) by women in all areas of the UK.

To conclude, it is clear that, in keeping with existing national and international research, women emerge as higher users of secondary care services (hospitals, nursing homes and social care homes) in the physical health sector in the UK than men. The trend is well established and holds for all parts of the UK. However, it is also clear from recent research on gender inequalities in health, especially the work of American sociologist Ingrid Waldron, that other factors, including age and marital status, need to be studied in order to understand the complexity of the relationship between gender and health. In the next two chapters, these factors will be explored more fully in the form of case-studies challenging commonly-held assumptions about the impact of marriage and age on physical health and illness.

Summary

- Life expectancy for women is at least five years longer than that for men
- The main causes of death in men are cardio-vascular diseases, cancers and accidents
- The main causes of death in women are breast cancer and cancers of the genito-urinary system
- Women are higher users of health services than men
- Women now dominate the population in residential health and social care facilities throughout the UK – outnumbering men by a ratio of 2.5 : 1
- Within the UK, Northern Ireland has the highest rate of bed occupancy in residential health and social care facilities. It also has a higher proportion of men in this population than either Scotland or England and Wales

5 Marriage is Good for Health

Chapter outline

- Introduction
- Examining the literature on marriage and health
- Theoretical perspectives on marriage and health
- Marriage and health – the impact of gender
- Health service use – the benefits of marriage
- Marriage and health service use – does gender make a difference?
- Gender, marriage and health service use – the mediating effect of age
- Summary

Introduction

Traditionally, marriage has been seen as the central institution in legitimising and regulating sex in almost all societies. It was regarded not only as the norm for most people but also as a permanent arrangement. Couples were expected to stay together – in good times and in bad, for richer and poorer, in sickness and in health – throughout their lives. Church leaders, politicians and social analysts defended the permanency of marriage by pointing to its economic and psychological benefits for both the individual and society. However, this view of marriage has been increasingly challenged in modern western society. Undermined internally by the sex-role revolution and externally by the rise of non-traditional family living patterns, such as co-habitation and single/never married parenthood, the institution of marriage no longer holds prime position as the best way of defining sexual relationships. Thus, in spite of its positive image in the past, marriage is no longer regarded as either a preferred or permanent way of life by an increasing number of people.

Questions arise, therefore, in relation to the impact of the changing position of marriage on other aspects of life – for example, on health. If marriage has lost its central role in society, has it also lost some of the benefits associated with it – economic prosperity and good health? It is with this question in mind that the following case-study investigates the population using residential health and social care services in the UK in the final three decades of the twentieth century. As in earlier discussions, the data for this case study are derived from an analysis of census data on occupants of all health and social care beds in health and social care facilities during this time period. Based on the premise that healthy people are low users or non-users of these services, we look at the relationship between marital status, gender and physical health. Using two theoretical perspectives – the 'marriage selection' and the 'marriage protection' hypotheses – we examine health differences between the married and non-married in the cared-for population, as well as differences both within and between male and female sub-populations in each marital category.

Marriage and health – the debate

The health benefits of marriage have been consistently confirmed in both national and international research (for comprehensive reviews of this literature, see Waldron *et al.*, 1996; Wyke and Ford, 1992). This is the particularly the case in the USA, where the most comprehensive studies have been carried out. In other words, all the evidence points to a positive relationship between marriage and health, irrespective of the focus of the research. Included in this research are studies of marital status and mortality (see Hu and Goldman, 1990; Gove, 1973), marital status and morbidity (see Verbrugge, 1979, 1989) and, to a lesser extent, marital status and health service use (see Morgan, 1980). Married people have lower mortality rates (they live longer), lower morbidity rates (they have fewer health problems/illnesses) and they are lower users of health services, than are their non-married counterparts. This is not to suggest, however, that all married people are equally healthy or that all non-married people are equally unhealthy. Within the non-married population, for example, there are identifiable differences between people who never married and those who were previously married (divorced, separated, or widowed). Although there are some exceptions, the general thrust of research findings in the UK, the USA and elsewhere in Europe is that people who never married are healthier than those who were previously married (Gijsbers van Wijk *et al.*, 1995; Wyke and Ford, 1992; Verbrugge, 1979).

Theoretical perspectives on marriage and health

A range of explanations for marital differences in the experience of good or bad health, and in the use of health services, has been put forward. These have been summarised in the research literature as 'marriage selection' and 'marriage protection' effects (see Waldron *et al.*, 1997, 1996; Wyke and Ford, 1992; Verbrugge, 1979).

Box 5.1 Theoretical explanations for the relationship between marriage and health

- The 'marriage selection' hypothesis
- The 'marriage protection' hypothesis

Focusing initially on the 'marriage selection' hypothesis, previous studies confirming this hypothesis tend to be of two kinds. Some compared the health status of individuals before they married – matching their health status with the decision to marry or not to marry. Others examined rates of marriage within populations with chronic illnesses or disabilities. Overall, the studies found that healthy people are more likely to get married than are unhealthy or disabled people. They also found that if less healthy or disabled people do marry, they are less likely to maintain their marriages and, thus, are more likely to be separated or divorced later in life. In other words, according to this perspective, there is a selection factor at work in relation to marriage that not only selects out less healthy individuals before marriage, but also continues to do so after a marriage has taken place. As Wyke and Ford (1992: 523), in summarising this relationship between marriage and health, conclude: 'marital status is seen to be dependent upon health'.

The 'marriage protection' hypothesis, in contrast, focuses on factors related to marriage that influence health behaviour or have a positive impact on experiences of illness. Arguing that health is dependent on marriage, proponents of this perspective suggest that marriage provides a protective shield that benefits all married people, regardless of age, gender, or ethnic origin. For example, marriage provides stability in that married people are believed to be less likely than non-married people to indulge in risk behaviours, such as excessive smoking and drinking, unhealthy diet or promiscuous sex. In addition, marriage is believed to protect people from stress by providing stable social roles and supportive relationships. Furthermore, it often brings with it economic benefits that impact positively on the individual's health. Even in the event of ill health, married people, it is suggested, have more support (practical and emotional) than those who are not married and, therefore, have a higher chance of recovery from illness or injury (for discussion, see Verbrugge, 1979).

It is important to remember when considering these views that, while either of these perspectives may be used as a direct explanation to account for the fact that married people have better health than those who are not married, they can also be used as an indirect explanation for health differences within the non-married population. For example, when the previously married and never married are compared, according to the 'marriage selection' perspective, it is the never married – people who have been selected out of marriage on the grounds of poor health – who are more likely to experience illnesses. An identical, but converse, pattern emerges when the 'marriage protection' hypothesis is considered. According to this perspective, it is the previously married, rather than the never married, that are more likely to experience poor health. Two reasons are given for this. Firstly, because divorced people may be de-selected out of marriage on the grounds of poor health, it is not unreasonable to assume that their original health status was probably similar to that of the never married – not good. Secondly, in contrast to their never married counterparts, the previously married have to contend with the additional stress caused by the break-up of a marriage due to divorce or the death of a spouse. According to this second perspective, it is these two factors – de-selection from marriage and the negative impact of the break-up of a marriage – in combination with a third factor – the loss of the protective benefits of marriage – that leaves previously married people more vulnerable to illness than never married people. This conclusion is supported by research on health differences within the non-married population. In other words, most of the evidence suggests that previously married people are likely to be less healthy than never married people (see Waldron *et al.*, 1996, 1997; Hu and Goldman, 1990; Verbrugge, 1979).

Gender, marriage and health

When gender is added to the equation, some inconsistent differences emerge in the relationship between marital status and health. For example, early research indicated that among men, mortality and morbidity rates for both groups of the non-married (never married and previously married) were similarly high in relation to the married group. However, this was not the case for women. Previously married women showed much higher rates of both mortality and morbidity than either married or never married women (Verbrugge, 1979). These and later research findings were interpreted as meaning that marriage was more beneficial for men than for women (House *et al.*, 1988; Macintyre, 1986). However, research by Mookherjee (1997) on perceptions of well-being, and by Kohler Riessman and Gerstel (1985) on morbidity rates, do not support this view. Mookherjee (1997) found that 'marriage enhances perceptions of well being for both men and women' and that women reported higher levels of satisfaction with marriage than did men. Kohler Riessman and Gerstel (1985) found that it was differences in other factors, such as type of health problem and the stage of dissolution of the marriage, and not marriage *per se*, that explained the better health status of previously married men as compared to that of previously married women.

As we saw in Chapter 1, general theoretical explanations for the seemingly contradictory trends in the relationship between gender and health have focused on differences in biological make-up, in social and economic roles and in health reporting behaviour. It is clear that many of these factors are affected by marital status. Current research on the impact of marriage on health emphasises the need to make a distinction between the impact of marriage *per se* and that of other factors, some of which are highly co-related to marriage (income, lifestyle and social support) and others not (employment, ethnicity, age). An example of this type of research is that of Waldron *et al.* (1997, 1996) on women's health in the USA. They found that the protective effects of marriage were significant only among women who were not employed. They also found that the differences between never married and previously married women were not consistent, but varied by age and cohort:

> Evidence from the 1970s and 1980s suggests that, among older women, divorced and separated women may have experienced more harmful health effects than never married women: however, among younger women, this difference may have been absent or possibly reversed. (Waldron *et al.*, 1997: 1387)

Another example, this time from the UK, is the study by Wyke and Ford (1992) on a sample of 55-year-old men and women in the West of Scotland. Their main finding was that good health among married men and women alike could be linked to higher levels of material resources and lower levels of stress – both characteristics more often associated with marriage than non-marriage. In other words, it may not be marriage in itself, but rather its associated advantages, that have a positive effect on health among both men and women.

In summary, then, empirical evidence suggests that, both directly and indirectly, marriage is beneficial for health. Irrespective of whether men or women are considered, married people demonstrate lower mortality and morbidity rates and they are also lower users of health services than are their non-married coun-terparts. However, as pointed out earlier, this does not mean that all married people are equally healthy or that all non-married people are equally unhealthy. Within the married population, for example, there is some empirical evidence to suggest identifiable differences between men and women. This is also the case when the never married and the previously married populations are compared, although the consensus of opinion is that people who never married are generally healthier than those who were pre-viously married.

To investigate this complex issue further, the following case study focuses on the relationship between gender, marriage and physical health in the UK. Using census data, it investigates health service use within the secondary care sector (for physical illness and disability) during the last three decades of the twentieth century. Based on the premise that healthy people are, for the most part, low users or non-users of these services, it examines differences in service use between the married and non-married in this population throughout the UK for the years 1971, 1981 and 1991. In addition, it also examines differences in health service use within the UK, both within and between male and female sub-populations, in each marital category in 1991.

Health service use – the benefits of marriage

Our case study confirms the positive relationship between mar-riage and physical health in the UK (see Table 5.1). In keeping with previous national and international research (Wyke and Ford, 1992; Hu and Goldman, 1990; Morgan, 1980; Gove, 1973), married people in the UK are much healthier than non-married people (the widowed, divorced and single/never married). As the data in Table 5.1 clearly show, when the married and the non-married were compared, married individuals demonstrated much lower occupancy levels in residential health and social care facil-ities in the three last decades of the twentieth century than did their non-married counterparts. In other words, the evidence from the secondary care sector suggests that married people were much healthier than non-married people. This health advantage increased dramatically during the 1970s and has been maintained

Table 5.1 Marital differences among bed occupants aged 15 years and over in physical health and social care facilities in the UK, 1971–91

	1971 (%)	1981 (%)	1991 (%)
Married	29.3	9.3	10.3
Non-Married	70.7	90.7	89.7
Widowed	(42.2)	(56.1)	(55.3)
Divorced	(1.1)	(1.9)	(2.5)
Single	(27.4)	(32.7)	(31.9)
Total	100.0	100.0	100.0
N	419,896	289,999	507,428

Source: England & Wales, Scotland, and Northern Ireland Census, 1971, 1981, 1991.

since then, so that by 1991 married people represented only 10 per cent of the total population in health and social care facilities in the UK. More importantly, however, this low level of health service use by married people occurred despite their continuing majority position in the total adult UK population – although this position did decline from 67 per cent in 1971 to 57 per cent in 1991 (Prior and Hayes, 2001c). Thus, in terms of the arguments presented at the beginning of this chapter, it is clear that marriage continues to be 'good' for the health of the UK population, in spite of the fact that it appears to be declining in popularity.

Within the non-married population, the previously married (widowed and divorced) showed much poorer health than the single/never married, as demonstrated by their much higher bed occupancy levels. This suggests that the 'marriage protection' hypothesis provides a better explanation of the relationship between marriage and health than the 'marriage selection' hypothesis. The poorest health seems to be linked to the loss of the marriage relationship, rather than to the lack of it, a finding that is in keeping with research in both the UK and the USA

(Wyke and Ford, 1992; Verbrugge, 1979). Among the previously married, we see that widowed people have consistently shown the poorest health. In 1991, widowed people formed over half (55 per cent) of the population in residential health and social care facilities in the UK, a trend that shows signs of continuing. This is in direct contrast to divorced people, who formed a very small, although increasing, proportion of this population since 1971 – reaching only 2.5 per cent in 1991.

When the census data were analysed more fully for England and Wales, we found that the widowed population in health and social care beds had increased steadily throughout the century – from 23 per cent in 1921 to 56 per cent in 1991 (see Prior and Hayes, 2002). More importantly, however, this dramatic increase in the widowed population in health and social care facilities occurred against a background of little change in the demographic composition of this group in the general population. For example, the widowed constituted just eight per cent of the total adult population in England and Wales in 1921, and have increased only marginally since then to nine per cent. The equivalent figures for the divorced in the general population were just one per cent or less until 1971, rising to four per cent in 1981, and increasing further to six per cent in 1991. This suggests that it is the death of a partner rather than divorce that seems to have the more negative effect on health. However, this finding requires further exploration in the future, as there may be other factors at work, the most probable being age.

In summary, then, the results of this analysis confirm the positive physical health benefits of marriage in the UK, in that married people are much lower users of residential health and social care services than the non-married. Furthermore, the positive health advantages of marriage hold in all parts of the UK – Scotland, England and Wales, and Northern Ireland (see Prior and Hayes, 2001c). This is not to deny, however, some important differences in the relationship between marital status and health across the UK. For example, whereas married people in Northern Ireland are at a much higher health risk than those in either Scotland or England and Wales, widowed people are at a much lower risk in Northern Ireland than elsewhere in the UK (Prior and Hayes, 2001c: 402). Northern Ireland also shows different patterns of bed occupancy among the non-married, with single/ never married people showing consistently higher levels than the widowed. These differences in the relationship between health and marriage between regions within the UK might be explained in terms of cultural differences in the position of marriage in society. Alternatively, they might be explained by different age patterns in the relevant populations. For example, the Northern Ireland population profile is younger than that of England and Wales [SSI (NI), 1998] – a fact that would impact on the number and proportion of widowed people both in the general population and in the population using secondary care services.

Marriage and health service use – are there gender differences?

As we have already seen, the international research literature shows that patterns of health and illness experienced by men are quite different from those experienced by women. Although there are exceptions to the trend (see Macintyre *et al.*, 1996), the most consistent pattern is that of higher morbidity (more illness) and lower mortality (longer life span) among women than men. Because of their longer life span, women tend to feature more prominently in morbidity statistics (including bed occupancy levels) than men. We also know that marriage impacts differently on men than on women and that, although it may be losing its position as a central institution in modern societies, it still continues to be a very powerful social force. In examining health data, therefore, we expect that gender differences will emerge in the relationship between marital status and health.

Is our expectation correct? In other words, are there differences between men and women in relation to marriage and health? Again, focusing on people in residential health and social care facilities, Table 5.2 addresses this question by examining marital differences in service use between men and women in the UK in 1991. Divided into separate panels for men (Panel A) and women (Panel B), this table shows the marital status of bed occupants within their respective male and female sub-

Table 5.2 The marital distribution of men and women aged 15 years and over in physical health and social care beds in the UK by region, 1991

	England & Wales (%)	Scotland (%)	Northern Ireland (%)	UK (%)
Panel A – Men				
Married	17.0	16.2	29.5	17.4
Non–Married	83.0	83.8	70.5	82.6
Widowed	(33.4)	(32.7)	(20.2)	(32.8)
Divorced	(4.8)	(3.7)	(2.1)	(4.6)
Single	(44.8)	(47.4)	(48.2)	(45.2)
Total	100.0	100.0	100.0	100.0
N	125,683	11,970	6,099	143,752
Panel B – Women				
Married	7.1	6.8	17.9	7.5
Non–Married	92.9	93.2	82.1	92.5
Widowed	(65.3)	(59.0)	(46.5)	(64.2)
Divorced	(1.8)	(1.1)	(1.0)	(1.7)
Single	(25.8)	(33.1)	(34.6)	(26.6)
Total	100.0	100.0	100.0	100.0
N	321,680	30,308	11,688	363,676

Source: England & Wales, Scotland, and Northern Ireland Census, 1991.

populations in England and Wales, Scotland, and Northern Ireland separately, as well as across the UK as a whole.

The first clear fact to emerge is that marriage is good for the health of both men and women – married men and married women are low users of residential health and social care services in all parts of the UK. As the data in Table 5.2 clearly shows, irrespective of whether men or women are considered, as a group, married people had much lower occupancy levels in residential health and social care facilities than their non-married counterparts. However, some very different gender patterns, or male-female differences, emerge in service use in all marital categories.

Comparing gender differences in the married population first, the most striking finding is that married men constitute a much larger proportion of the male sub-population in health and social care facilities than do married women in their equivalent female sub-population, in all areas of the UK. For example, whereas married men accounted for 17 per cent of the male sub-population in health and social care facilities throughout the UK in 1991, the equivalent figure among females was less than half that, at just eight per cent. It is important to note that this gender disparity in health service use among the married cannot be explained in terms of demographic patterns in the general population as a whole. For example, in 1991, while the proportion of married men in the adult male population in the UK was 60 per cent, the proportion of married women in the adult female population was only slightly lower at 55 per cent (Prior and Hayes, 2001c).

This finding seems to indicate that in the UK at the end of the twentieth century, marriage has proved more beneficial for the health of women than it has for the health of men. It, therefore, contradicts existing research, which found the opposite to be the case – that is, that marriage is more beneficial for men (House *et al.*, 1988; Macintyre, 1986). However, as will be shown in the next section, a key factor in explaining this unexpected finding is the disproportionate concentration of divorced and widowed individuals within the female sub-population, particularly among those aged 65 years and over. In other words, once age is added to the equation and the marital composition of men and women within their respective sub-populations is compared directly, the results of this study suggests that, in fact, marriage is of equal benefit to the health of men and women.

It is among non-married men and women, however, that some of the most interesting gender differences in the health benefits of marriage emerge. For example, whereas single/never married men emerge as the most vulnerable group within the non-married male sub-population, it is widows who are the most vulnerable within the non-married female sub-population. For example, whereas single/never married men accounted for almost half (45 per cent) of all males in residential health and social care facilities in the UK in 1991, the equivalent figure among females within their sub-population was much lower at just 27 per cent. This finding fits in with earlier research that has shown the greater vulnerability to illness of single/never married men, when compared with single/never married women (Waldron *et al.*, 1997; Wyke and Ford, 1992; Verbrugge, 1979). However, it also points to a much worse state of health for single/never married men in the UK in the 1990s than that reported elsewhere.

A similar gender pattern is echoed in the divorced population – with divorced men showing worse health than divorced women. For example in 1991, divorced men constituted five per cent of the male sub-population in residential health and social care facilities, while divorced women formed only two per cent of the female sub-population in the same facilities. In the widowed population, however, the gender pattern is reversed – with widowed females showing a much worse health profile than widowed males. For example, the proportion of widowers in the male sub-population in residential health and social care facilities in 1991 was almost half that of widows in the female sub-population – 33 per cent as compared with 64 per cent. Therefore, we can say that, among previously married people, for women the highest health risks are associated with widowhood, while for men they are associated with divorce. These patterns are consistent across all parts of the UK, although there are some interesting variations, as reflected in the greater concentration of widowed females in England and Wales and of both married males and females in Northern Ireland.

Gender and the health benefits of marriage – the importance of age

The importance of considering age in examining differences in the benefits of marriage has been emphasised in earlier research on gender and health (Waldron *et al.*, 1997; Macintyre, 1986; Verbrugge, 1979). As already discussed, research in the USA, for example, has shown that not only do the protective benefits of marriage differ between never married and previously married women, but also that these benefits vary by age and cohort. In other words, although older women who were divorced and separated experienced more ill health than never married women, among younger women, however, this difference appeared to be absent and, in some cases, reversed (Waldron *et al.*, 1997: 1387). The question we pose here is, 'To what extent are these gendered and age-specific marital differences in health also reflected in the UK population?'. To answer this question, we analysed the age distribution across marital groups for both men and women in residential health and social care facilities throughout the UK in 1991 (see Table 5.3). Similar patterns prevailed when each of its three constituent parts – England and Wales, Scotland, and Northern Ireland – were investigated separately (for a more detailed discussion, see Prior and Hayes, 2001c).

The results of this analysis suggest that, when the within-population age distributions are considered, there are substantial age-specific health differences in relation to gender among divorced and single people. Although married men and women are again healthier than the non-married, as reflected in their much lower and similar occupancy levels in health and social care facilities, among the non-married, however, the effect of gender is strongly mediated by age. In other words, although the overall pattern is the same for men and women – the non-married are less healthy than the married – some notable differences emerge among divorced and single people of working age (15 to 64 years). For example, while the proportion of divorced men under the age of 65 in the cared for population was notably higher than that for divorced women, this pattern was even more pronounced when single people were considered. In other words, in the working-age population, it is single men who have the poorest health. What this means is that the absence of marriage has a much greater negative impact on the health of working age men than it has on women of a similar age. Or to put it another way – marriage has a much more positive effect on men's health than on women's health.

This is not to deny, however, the similar health advantages of marriage for both men and women. As the results of our study show clearly, both married men and women are healthier than the non-married, as reflected in their much lower and almost

Table 5.3 The marital composition and age distribution of men and women aged 15 years and over in physical health and social care beds in the UK, 1991

Age	Married (%)	Widowed (%)	Divorced (%)	Single (%)
Panel A − Men				
Under 65 years	13.1	1.5	39.7	63.9
15–24	(0.3)	(0.0)	(0.4)	(12.4)
25–34	(1.9)	(0.0)	(3.5)	(16.6)
35–44	(2.5)	(0.1)	(9.0)	(13.6)
45–54	(2.4)	(0.1)	(10.1)	(10.8)
55–64	(6.0)	(1.3)	(16.7)	(10.5)
65 years and over	86.9	98.5	60.3	36.1
65–74	(19.0)	(11.5)	(30.5)	(15.5)
75–84	(43.8)	(44.0)	(23.9)	(14.9)
85+	(24.1)	(43.0)	(5.9)	(5.7)
Total	100.0	100.0	100.0	100.0
N	25,071	47,102	6,575	65,004
Panel B − Women				
Under 65 years	13.3	0.8	28.0	36.1
15–24	(0.9)	(0.0)	(0.4)	(10.4)
25–34	(2.9)	(0.0)	(3.3)	(8.4)
35–44	(2.1)	(0.0)	(5.6)	(6.3)
45–54	(2.3)	(0.1)	(6.1)	(5.3)
55–64	(5.1)	(0.7)	(12.6)	(5.7)
65 years and over	86.7	99.2	72.0	63.9
65–74	(16.8)	(7.0)	(25.8)	(10.7)
75–84	(42.5)	(38.2)	(30.9)	(23.9)
85+	(27.4)	(54.0)	(15.3)	(29.3)
Total	100.0	100.0	100.0	100.0
N	27,153	233,429	6,097	96,997

Source: England & Wales, Scotland, and Northern Ireland Census, 1991.

identical occupancy levels in health and social care facilities. Thus, contrary to our early findings – which suggested that the positive impact of marriage was a disproportionately female phenomenon – the results of this later analysis point to similar health advantages related to marriage for both men and women. What may explain this discrepancy in the findings? As previously suggested, a key factor in accounting for our earlier conclusion was the potentially distorting effect of a disproportionate concentration of divorced and widowed individuals within the female sub-population, particularly among those aged 65 years and over. The result of this later analysis confirms this interpretation. In other words, once age is added to the equation and the marital composition of men and women within their respective sub-populations is compared directly, it is clear that marriage is of equal benefit to the health of men and women.

In conclusion, this case study confirms research findings elsewhere, that marriage has a positive impact on health, by showing that married people form a very small proportion of the population in residential health and social care facilities throughout the UK. What is most interesting about this finding is that the positive effect of marriage on health has increased steadily since the 1970s, despite the challenges to marriage in modern society. The case study also confirms earlier research findings of substantial gender differences in health within the non-married population, suggesting that, within the working age population (15 to 64 years), the absence of marriage has a greater negative impact on the health of men than of women. Finally, it is clear that any research on gender differences in the experience of health and on health service use in the UK must take into account the important mediating influence of age. Not only does the dominance of women in the older population have a significant impact on health statistics – sometimes obscuring patterns of health and illness – but this is particularly the case when the married population is considered. In the next chapter, we look specifically at some of the issues arising from the relationship between age and health and its potential impact on future health provision.

Summary

- Existing research indicates that marriage is good for physical health and that it is more advantageous to the health of men than the health of women
- Married people are much lower users than are non-married people of secondary care services (for physical illness and disability) in the UK
- Within the non-married population, previously married people appear to have worse health than single/never married people in the UK
- When men and women are considered separately, married women appear to be much healthier than married men, as demonstrated by their much lower use of secondary care services in the UK
- Among the non-married population, whereas the single/never married emerge as the most vulnerable group among men, widows appear to have the poorest health among women
- Age is a very important mediating factor in any study of marriage and health. Although marriage is equally beneficial to men and women of all ages, in the working-age population the absence of marriage appears to be more damaging to the health of men than of women

6 Older Women are Most Vulnerable

Introduction

In common with the rest of the western industrialised world, the UK has an ageing population. In 1901, about one person in 20 was over the age of 65 and one in 100 was over the age of 75. By 1998, this increased to just over one in six for those over the age of 65 and one in fourteen for those over the age of 75. At the same time, the proportion of the population under the age of 16 fell from a third to just over a fifth. Demographic projections suggest that these trends will continue. For example, by 2011, it is predicted that the number of people over the age of 65 will be greater than the number under the age of 16 –

81

11.9 million as compared to 11.3 million – and the majority of dependants in the UK will be retired people (ONS, 2000a: 8).

This increase in the older population has been largest among women. Women currently begin to outnumber men from around the age of 50 and by the age of 89 there are about three women to every man. However, the most dramatic gender differences in survival rates have occurred among the 'very old' – people living to the age of 100. In 1911, women centenarians outnumbered men centenarians by about three to one, but by 1996, the rates had increased to eight to one. In other words, for every man who reached the age of 100 in the UK in 1996, there were eight women who had done so. While the number of centenarians is still fairly small – 5,500 in England and Wales in 1996 – the rate of increase since the beginning of the twentieth century has been very fast, roughly doubling every decade. Population projections suggest that by 2036, there could be over 40 thousand centenarians alive in England and Wales, the vast majority of whom will be women (ONS, 2000b: 25).

The question arises, therefore, of the impact of these changing demographic trends on health. In other words, has the growth in the older population led to a substantial rise in the number and proportion of people over the age of 65 using health and social care services? Furthermore, are older women more prominent in this respect than older men? It is with these two questions in mind that the following case study investigates the older population using residential health and social care services in the UK in the final three decades of the twentieth century. As in our previous case study, this information is derived from an analysis of census data on occupants of all 'general' health and social care beds during this time period. Using two competing perspectives – the 'increasing burden' versus the 'continuing independence' hypotheses – we examine age and gender differences in this institution-based population, as well as comparing age differences in living arrangements – private household versus care facility – within the older female sub-population as a whole.

Health care needs of older people – the debate

To date, two competing perspectives are clear in the arguments used to explain the future health care needs of older people. These have been presented in the research literature as the 'increasing burden' versus the 'continuing independence' hypothesis (see Lyons *et al.*, 1997; Ribbe *et al.*, 1997; Wilson, 2000). While both acknowledge that health standards have improved dramatically throughout the western world during the twentieth century, leading to longer lives for most people, they differ as to the actual consequences of this increasing longevity, particularly in relation to projected health care costs. For example, whereas proponents of the 'increasing burden' hypothesis stress the rapidly increasing health care costs of an ever-growing older population, advocates of the 'continuing independence' hypothesis reject this view as nothing more than an ill-informed and stereotypically-based mis-representation of the health care needs of older people.

Box 6.1 Competing perspectives on the health care needs of older people

• The 'increasing burden' hypothesis
• The 'continuing independence' hypothesis

We focus initially on the 'increasing burden' hypothesis, which emphasises the ever-increasing health care costs of older people. According to this perspective, not only does the ageing process result in poorer health for many people, but as people now live longer, they also make extra demands on a range of health services (see Lyons *et al.*, 1997; Ribbe *et al.*, 1997; DoH, 1996). In other words, older people are perceived not only as higher users of general health services than younger people, but also as higher users of very costly medical and nursing services at the end of their lives. Because of this perception, they are regarded as an increasing burden on society, especially in countries where the health care system is funded primarily from the public purse, as is the case in the UK. This growing fear of an impending finan-cial burden brought on by an ageing population is evident in the UK in the work of the Royal Commission on Long Term Care for the Elderly (Sutherland Report, 1999). It is also reflected in the endless policy discussions on the problems of funding current and future health and social care services for older people (for discussion, see Parker, 2000; Bernard and Phillips, 1998; Evandrou, 1997; Parker and Clarke, 1997).

However, there is an alternative view, or the 'continuing independence' hypothesis, as reflected in the work of Gail Wilson (2000: 8–15), a social policy researcher from the London School of Economics. Although admitting that the costs associated with ageing – such as a lengthy retirement period and the increased need for care – cannot be denied, Wilson argues that the moral panic and the 'doom and gloom' predictions based on these alleged costs are open to question. According to Wilson, much of the current debate, which stereotypes older people (and particularly older women) as an ever-expanding economic and social burden on younger people in society, is based on misrepresentations or misinterpretations of facts. In the health care arena, for example, she cites international evidence showing that, contrary to popular opinion, the highest costs for care consistently occur only in the last two to four years of life, regardless of the age at death (OECD, 1998). Furthermore, the rise in medical costs associated with an ageing population 'is much slower than the rise in total numbers of old people' (Wilson, 2000: 110) and 'acute care costs decrease as the elderly age' (Perls, 1997: 123). In other words, according to Wilson and Perls, the fact that people live longer does not necessarily mean that they will need care for longer or that the care will be costly. In fact the opposite may be true. If people become healthier due to changing health behaviour in earlier life they may need less care than previous generations and will be likely to continue to lead independent lives well into old age.

Mindful of these competing hypotheses, this case study focuses on the use of residential health and social care services by older people in the UK in the final three decades of the twentieth century. Specifically the research questions to be addressed are:

(1) Has there been a substantial rise in the number and proportion of people over the age of 65 using costly health services – in this instance, institution-based care?
(2) Are older women more burdensome than men in this respect?
(3) Finally, what is the balance of residential care provision for older women between the health sector and the social care sector?

By answering these questions, we hope to present a coherent statistical picture of the present and future health needs of older people in the UK – with a special focus on women. This information is invaluable at this particular time for two reasons. First, a review of the literature suggests that current debates on the health costs of an ageing population in the UK have been based on extremely scanty empirical evidence (for discussion, see Arber and Cooper, 1999). Second, given demographic projections as to the importance of the late twentieth century as a crucial turning point in the accelerated rise of the 'very old' female population, any information related to the present position will provide an important benchmark for future planning and research.

The impact of ageing on health

Turning now to the results, the first finding from our case study lends support to the 'increasing burden' hypothesis, in that ageing has a substantial negative effect on health. As the data in Figure 6.1 clearly show, as a group, older people (aged 65 years and over) are much higher users of secondary care services in the UK than

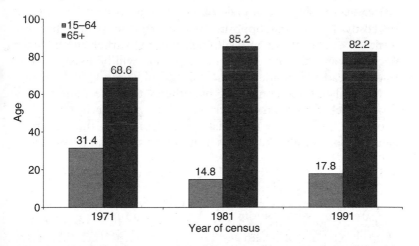

Figure 6.1 The growth in the older population in physical health and social care facilities in the UK, 1971–91

Source: England & Wales, Scotland, Northern Ireland Census, 1971, 1981, 1991.

their younger counterparts (aged 18–64 years). In 1981, for example, people aged 65 years or older outnumbered those aged under 65 years in health and social care facilities by a ratio of almost 6 to 1. Although the proportion of older people in these facilities decreased slightly in 1991, the number of older people as a percentage of the population in health and social care beds in the UK rose by 13 points – from 69 per cent to 82 per cent – between 1971 and 1991.

It is important to note, however, that this percentage increase occurred in the context of an overall rise in the population in health and social care facilities – from 419,896 in 1971 to 507,428 in 1991 – or a net increase of 87,532 individuals. In other words, as the total population in these facilities increased, so too did the proportion of older people in them. In contrast to the working-age population, which experienced a net decrease of 41,246 people in residential health and social care facilities between these two time periods, the number of those aged 65 years or older rose from 288,161 in 1971 to 416,939 in 1991 – a net increase of 128,778 people. It appears, in addition, that the overall trend was not affected by the reduction in the number of bed occupants between 1971 and 1981 – from 419,896 to 289,999 – caused by an increasing use of day-surgery and day-care (see discussion in Chapter 3). Rather, this change in medical practice also served to further reduce the working-age population (under 65 years) in favour of the retired population within these facilities.

A gendered service

When we compare the number of men and women using secondary care services in the UK, the gendered nature of service use becomes clear. As discussed earlier, current research on gender and health highlights two facts that are important in the discussion here – firstly, that women live an average of five years longer than men and, secondly, that women tend to have higher levels of morbidity and of health service use than men. With these facts in mind, we explore the relationship between gender and age in the population using residential health and social care services in

Table 6.1 Gender differences among older people in physical health and social care facilities in the UK, 1971–91

Age	Men (%)			Women (%)		
	1971	1981	1991	1971	1981	1991
15–64	38.2	22.9	33.5	28.0	11.9	11.6
65+	61.8	77.1	66.5	72.0	88.1	88.4
N	138,702	74,511	143,752	281,194	215,488	363,676

Source: England & Wales, Scotland, and Northern Ireland Census, 1971, 1981, 1991.

the UK. If we look at Table 6.1, we see that there are three clear gender patterns in this population, two of which have already emerged in our earlier analysis.

The first is that, as expected, women are higher users of residential health and social care services than men. In 1991, there were 363,676 women as opposed to 143,752 men in the cared-for population. The second finding is that the female sub-population has a much older age profile than the male sub-population in these facilities. In 1991, for example, while older women (65 years and over) constituted 88 per cent of the female cared-for population, older men formed only 67 per cent of the male cared-for population. The third finding is the differing rates at which the proportion of elderly occupants increased within their respective male and female sub-populations. In other words, not only does the female sub-population have a much older profile than the male sub-population in these facilities, but the increase among older women (65 years and over) was much faster than the increase among older men. For example, while the pro-portion of older women within the female sub-population rose from 72 per cent in 1971 to 88 per cent in 1991 – an increase of 16 percentage points – the equivalent growth among older men within the male sub-population was much lower, at just five per cent. More importantly, however, this disproportionate and faster growth among the elderly within the female sub-population translated into a numerical increase of 118,881 women – 202,456 in 1971 as compared to 321,337 in 1991 – in these facilities as compared to a net increase of just 9,897 men of an equivalent age.

There is no doubt, therefore, that this case study lends strong support to the 'increasing burden' hypothesis, or the dispropor- tionate increase in the use of secondary care services by older people in the UK. It also further confirms existing research find- ings of a substantial increase in the numbers of older women using these health and social care services at the end of the twentieth century (see also Arber and Cooper, 1999; Arber, 1997; Ribbe *et al.*, 1997). This is not to deny the increasing presence of older men in this cared-for population, though on a much smaller scale. It is important to note, however, that this increase in the use of secondary care services among older women cannot be understood as simply a by-product of their greater and increas- ing longevity within the UK population as a whole. Additional analysis, again using census data, confirms that although the total number of older (aged 65 years or over) women in the UK population increased by 18 per cent during this time period – from just under four-and-a-half million in 1971 to over five million in 1991 – the equivalent rise among older women in sec- ondary care facilities – from 202,456 in 1971 to 321,337 in 1991 – was significantly higher at 59 per cent. In other words, the rate of increase among older women in the cared-for population was over five times the size of their increase in the general popula- tion in the UK, during the same time period.

Independence versus care

Although our earlier analysis within the secondary care sector lends support to the 'increasing burden' hypothesis, particularly in the case of older women, a further analysis, dividing the total UK older female population according to place of residence, casts serious doubt on this interpretation. In other words, when the total older (aged 65 years and over) female population is sub-divided in terms of specific living arrangements – private household versus care facility – we find that an overwhelming majority of older women continue to live independently. As

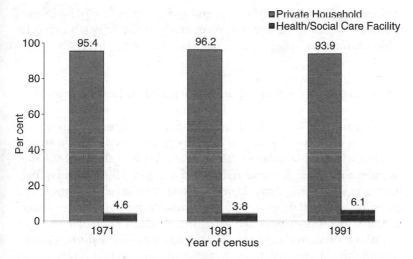

Figure 6.2 Differences in residential patterns among women aged 65 years and over in the UK, 1971–91

Source: England & Wales, Scotland, Northern Ireland Census, 1971, 1981, 1991.

the data in Figure 6.2 clearly show, most older women in the UK live in private households and not in residential health and social care facilities. For example, 95 per cent of women aged 65 years or older lived in private households in 1971, a proportion that had reduced only slightly, to 94%, between 1981 and 1991.

This finding is consistent with international research, which suggests that '90–95 per cent of elders remain at home, with many of them receiving formal and informal support services' (Ribbe et al., 1997: 7). However, although the vast majority of older women continue to live independently, there are also substantial numbers receiving institution-based care – 321,337 in 1991, or 6 per cent of the total female population over the age of 65 years. This use of residential health and social care facilities by older women has already made a huge impact on these services. As explained earlier, not only has it led to an expansion in the overall size of the cared-for population but it has also resulted in two distinct changes in the pattern of service use within existing provision. The gender-related impact has been that beds occupied by men in the past are now occupied by older women, while the age-related impact has been that beds occupied by people of working-age (men and women) in the past are now occupied by older women.

The mediating effect of age on independent living

As explained previously, although there is general agreement among social scientists and policy analysts that dramatic improvements in health standards have increased the life-span of most people, the actual consequences of this increasing longevity, particularly in terms of the health profile among older people, are open to dispute. For example, advocates of the 'increasing burden' hypothesis simply stress the increasing health care needs of older people, irrespective of their specific age profile. Advocates of the 'continuing independence' hypothesis, in contrast, reject this blanket view and point to important age-specific distinctions within the older population in terms of their health care requirements. In other words, not only do supporters of the latter position stress the continuing independence of many older individuals, but this is particularly the case when the 'young-old', or individuals aged under 75 years, are considered (for discussion, see Wilson, 2000).

To what extent, are these age-specific differences in health care needs also evident in the older female population in the UK? To address this question, Table 6.2 presents the age profiles divided into six mutually exclusive age-bands for the retired female population in terms of their place of residence – private household versus care facility – in the UK for the last three decades of the twentieth century. To distinguish between private households and care facilities, the table is divided into two panels. Panel A, which presents the age profiles for women aged 65 years or over in private households, and Panel B, which shows the equivalent age-specific data for women in health and social care facilities. It is clear from Table 6.2 that the expansion in numbers of older women in institution-based care has not been caused by a trend towards a loss of independence earlier in life. In fact, the opposite is the case – many women are living independently for longer. This is not to deny, however, the dramatic growth in the

Table 6.2 Age differences in residential patterns among women aged 65 years and over in the UK, 1971–91

	Year of Census		
Age	1971 (%)	1981 (%)	1991 (%)
Panel A: Private household			
65–69	34.9	31.5	29.5
70–74	28.0	28.0	25.0
75–79	19.3	20.9	21.5
80–84	11.4	12.4	14.7
85–89	4.9	7.2	7.0
90+	1.5	—	2.3
Total	100.0	100.0	100.0
N	4,211,792	4,769,790	4,909,253
Panel B: Health or social care facility			
65–69	9.0	4.3	3.6
70–74	13.7	9.0	6.6
75–79	18.9	17.5	14.1
80–84	24.8	25.8	25.1
85–89	20.8	24.6	28.2
90+	12.8	18.8	22.4
Total	100.0	100.0	100.0
N	202,456	189,722	321,337

Note: Individuals living in private households aged between 85 and 89 years and those 90 years or above could not be distinguished in the 1981 census.

Source: England & Wales, Scotland, and Northern Ireland Census, 1971, 1981, 1991.

number of older women – particular those aged 85 years or older – as users of secondary care services.

Focusing initially on older women living independently in private households, or Panel A in Table 6.2, we see that in 1971, only 37 per cent of women over the age of 75 were living in private households. By 1991, however, this proportion had increased to 46 per cent. In other words, although the majority of the older female population living independently – in private households – are aged between 65 and 74 years, since 1971, there has also been a notable increase in the proportion of women over the age of 75 in this population. Between 1971 and 1991 the proportion of women in this age category increased by nine percentage points – from 37 per cent in 1971 to 46 per cent in 1991.

When we look at the female population in residential health and social care facilities, we see the other side of the same coin (see Panel B). Here, the proportion of women aged 65–84 years decreased by 17 per cent – from 66 per cent to 49 per cent – between 1971 and 1991. The steepest age-specific drop happened among 70–74 year olds, among whom the proportion halved – from 14 per cent in 1971 to 7 per cent in 1991. This is in direct contrast to women aged 90 years and older, who showed the greatest increase in the cared-for population over this time period. This age group almost doubled in the 20-year period as a proportion of the over-65-year-old female population in care – from 13 per cent in 1971 to 22 per cent in 1991 – reflecting a dramatic increase in numerical terms, from 25,822 to 71,941. When the numbers for the next oldest age group are added to this, the scale of this increase among the 'very old' becomes even more apparent. When the two age bands are combined, the actual number of women aged 85 years and over in health and social care beds more than doubled – from 67,992 in 1971 to 162,690 in 1991 – or a net increase of 94,698 women, between these two time periods.

These findings are consistent with existing research and confirm that improved health standards in the general population also extend into old age (Baggott, 1998: 11). However, the increase in the number of women over the age of 80 years in the general population has led to a much higher use of secondary care services by this specific group. Policy literature on the health care needs of older people often distinguishes between the 'younger old' and the 'older old' – those aged under 75 years versus those aged over 75 years – as a crude categorisation of health and well-being. The 'younger old' are assumed to be healthy and, therefore, low users of health and social care services, while the 'older old' are assumed to be less healthy and, therefore, more dependent on these services. The results of this analysis suggests, however, that this categorisation is open to challenge because the age at which people move into the 'older old' category, in terms of their health care needs, is rising continually.

Therefore, it may be concluded that the largest increase in the population of older women in health and social care facilities, during this period, was among the 'older old' – those aged 85 years and older – rather than among the 'younger old' – those aged 65–84 years. In other words, the need for institution-based care is increasingly concentrated in the female population over the age of 85 years. This finding further strengthens the argument that the threshold between the 'healthy younger old' and the 'unhealthy older old' is moving upwards – in this case the watershed seems to be 85 years of age, which is older than reported in the past (for discussion, see Phillipson, 1998). Thus, it seems that the increasing presence of older women in residential health and social care facilities in the UK has much more to do with the longer life-span enjoyed by women than it has with other factors, such as the dissolution of family networks. Women are living independently for longer than ever before, but, as the average life-span of women increases, there will inevitably be women over the age of 85, who will require care. This is mainly due to the fact that, by that age, they will have lost the support of their male partners and many of their siblings. It is also exacerbated by the increasing geographical mobility of the younger generations.

Health or social care?

Having established the fact that older women do, indeed, form the majority of the population in health and social care facilities in the UK, and that their numbers are increasing, particularly

Table 6.3 Age differences by sector among women aged 65 years and over in residential health and social care facilities in the UK, 1971–91

Age	1971 (%)	1981 (%)	1991 (%)
Panel A – Health sector (hospitals and nursing homes)			
65–69	13.0	5.2	9.5
70–74	16.4	10.0	11.5
75–79	19.6	17.7	16.4
80–84	22.6	25.0	22.5
85–89	17.5	22.9	22.7
90+	10.9	19.2	17.4
Total	100.0	100.0	100.0
N	92,354	46,798	26,555
Panel B – Social care sector (care homes)			
65–69	5.6	4.1	3.1
70–74	11.3	8.7	6.2
75–79	18.4	17.4	13.8
80–84	26.7	26.0	25.3
85–89	23.6	25.1	28.8
90+	14.4	18.7	22.8
Total	100.0	100.0	100.0
N	110,102	142,924	294,782

Source: England & Wales, Scotland, and Northern Ireland Census, 1971, 1981, 1991.

among those aged over 85, the question remains as to which sector – health or social care – has witnessed the greatest expansion in provision. To address this question, Table 6.3 presents the age profile of the retired female population in secondary care in the UK in terms of two distinct sectors – the health sector and the social care sector. As discussed in Chapter 1, secondary care facilities include the complete range of providers (public, commercial and non-profit) in two distinct sectors. These are the health sector – consisting of general hospitals and nursing homes – and the social care sector – consisting of residential facilities for older people (including facilities for physical disability). In this case study, this distinction between the two sectors is maintained, that is, the health sector includes all hospitals and nursing homes, and the social care sector includes all residential care facilities.

As can be seen in Table 6.3, the age trends are similar in both sectors – a decrease in the proportion of women under the age of 85 and an increase in the proportion of women over that age – particular among those aged 90 years or older – since 1971. However, the two sectors are quite different in terms of patterns of service use, and these differences are growing. While the number of older women in the health sector (hospitals and nursing homes) has plummeted since 1971, the opposite has been the case in the social care sector (residential care facilities). Two specific facts are very important. The first is that the size of the population of women in the social care sector almost trebled between 1971 and 1991 – from 110,102 to 294,782. The second is that the gap in the level of provision between the two sectors has widened to such an extent that the social care sector now provides approximately 90 per cent of all care for older women. This is due not only to the growth in the female population in social care facilities, but also to a decrease in the female population in the health sector (hospitals and nursing homes) – from 92,354 in 1971 to 26,555 in 1991.

This last finding fits with existing evidence on the fall in bed numbers for older people within NHS structures since the 1970s (Parker, 2000: 136; Hensher and Edwards, 1999). It is also in keeping with existing evidence of the growth in commercially-run social care facilities during the 1980s. This was due to the perverse incentive, which existed within the UK social security system for a brief period, allowing older people (and people with disabilities) to seek admission to residential or nursing care in the first instance and later apply for a subsidy to cover the cost of care. This perverse incentive may be summarised as follows. Because social security staff could not assess people on their need for care, but only on their income, most people received the subsidy, which was paid directly to the nursing or residential home. Because of the relative ease with which individuals could get funding for residential and nursing care, the private sector responded by expanding the number of places available in nursing homes and social care homes. This, in turn, led to an increase in the population in these facilities (for discussion, see Parker, 2000). This incentive was removed through the *NHS and Community Care Act, 1990*, which made public funding for care available only after an assessment by social services staff on the need for care. As a result of this, a slowing down in the rate of increase in the population in social care facilities might be expected during the early 1990s – a trend which will only be verifiable after the data from the 2001 census are released. For the moment, however, it is clear that any bids for funds targeted at the care of older people must take into consideration the vital importance of the social care sector. This sector now provides approximately 90 per cent of all institution-based care for older women.

In conclusion, then, in this chapter we have explored one of the most pervasive stereotypical notions held in relation to age and gender in the use of health services – that older people are high users of costly health services and that women predominate within this group. The data provided by the census on occupants of health and social care beds in the UK in the last thirty years of the twentieth century, show that this notion is only partially true. The number of older people who are users of secondary care services is indeed increasing both proportionately and numerically and women are in the majority. However, the services being used are not in the expensive health sector (hospital and nursing homes) but in the 'economy' social care sector (residential facilities), which has a low level of medical and nursing input. More importantly, however, the vast majority of older women live independently in private households. In the UK, as in many western countries (Ribbe *et al.*, 1997), between 94 and 95 per cent of all older women live at home. Furthermore, the proportion of women living independently, who are over the age of 75 years, has been increasing steadily during the past thirty years, a trend that seems set to continue.

Summary

- By 2011 in the UK, the number of people over the age of 65 will be greater than the number under the age of 16. Women will be in the majority in this older population
- Older people (65 years and over) form the majority of the population in residential health (hospitals and nursing homes) and social care facilities in the UK
- Older women have poorer health than older men, as demonstrated by their higher use of residential health and social care
- The majority of older women continue to live independently in private households, with only 6 per cent requiring care
- Women are living independently for longer – with those over the age of 85 years being most likely to require residential care
- Approximately 90 per cent of all institution-based care for women in the UK is in the social care sector

Part III
Stereotypes Rejected?

7 Gender and Mental Health

Introduction

Gender differences in the experience of mental disorder and in the use of mental health services have been the subject of intensive academic research and debate throughout the western world (for reviews of the literature, see Prior, 1999; Busfield, 1994, 1996). The historical origins of this debate can be found in medical writings in the seventeenth century. At that time, Dr Richard Napier suggested that women patients were twice as likely as men to show signs of mental disorder (MacDonald, 1981). This pattern was confirmed in the writings of the

Scottish alienist Dr. W. A. F. Browne, who proposed that 'in the case of a public asylum, a larger proportion of the building should be allotted to females, as their numbers almost always predominate' (Browne, 1837, reprinted in Scull, 1991: 184). During that period – the eighteenth and nineteenth centuries – it was generally assumed that women were 'madder' than men. In modern times, the pattern of female dominance in mental health statistics has continued throughout the western world (see Dennerstein, 1995; Pilowsky *et al.*, 1991; Gove and Tudor, 1973).

It is interesting to note, however, that this predominance of women in mental health statistics is not a universal finding. For example, in the mid-nineteenth century, an American physician, Edward Jarvis, suggested that men were more prone to insanity than women, based on his analysis of reports from 250 hospitals in America and Europe (Jarvis, 1850, cited in Dohrenwend, 1975: 368). In Ireland, men predominated as patients in the public asylum system throughout the nineteenth century, a pattern that continues to the present day in the Republic of Ireland (see Cleary, 1997; Finnane, 1981). In New Zealand, similarly, there is a higher level of reported psychiatric morbidity among men than among women (Thornley *et al.*, 1991). This is not to deny, however, the well-established pattern of female dominance in most mental health statistics throughout the western world. In other words, as a group, women shown significantly higher levels of psychiatric morbidity and mental health service use than men.

In recent years, however, a growing body of empirical literature has emerged that suggests a possible reversal in this trend. During the 1990s, for example, not only have a range of American studies demonstrated a substantial rise in levels of psychiatric morbidity and mental health service use among men, but this is also increasingly the case in Britain (Payne, 1995, 1996; Meltzer *et al.*, 1995; Kessler *et al.*, 1994; Robins and Regier, 1991). This growing visibility of men in mental health statistics – most notably young men – has begun to cast serious doubt on the assumption of women as the 'madder sex'. It is with these recent empirical findings in mind that we focus, in Part III, on gender differences in mental health statistics, and on the gendered nature of psychiatric service use within the UK.

The mental health of women

In the early 1970s, Gove and Tudor (1973) documented the dominance of women in community psychiatric morbidity surveys, in first admissions to mental hospitals, in treatment by psychiatrists, and in psychiatric treatment in general hospitals. The research findings from these earlier studies are confirmed in current psychiatric statistics – women are high users of all mental health services, far outstripping men. The main diagnoses associated with women are depression and neurosis, affecting large sections of the population. Other well-known diagnoses include anorexia nervosa and bulimia nervosa. Though highly publicised, these eating disorders have very low incidence rates except among adolescent girls in western societies. In contrast, about one in five women are estimated to suffer from depression at some time in their lives.

The best examples of these findings from American mental health research come from the Epidemiologic Catchment Area (ECA) Survey and the National Co-Morbidity Survey (NCS). The ECA, a major study with 18,571 participants was carried out in the 1980s in five areas of the USA (Regier *et al.*, 1993). This study found that women had higher yearly and lifetime prevalence rates than men for all symptoms of depression (Robins and Regier, 1991: 63, 68). Similarly the NCS – another major survey undertaken in the early 1990s on a nationally representative sample of 8,098 people – reported that women had a one-year prevalence of 14 per cent for any affective disorder (major depressive episode, manic episode and dysthymia), while for men it was 9 per cent. The greatest gender difference was for major depression, with women almost twice as likely as men to report at least one depressive episode in their lives – a lifetime prevalence of 21 per cent for women as compared to just 13 per cent for men (Kessler *et al.*, 1994: 13).

Women are also found in greater numbers in statistics on neurosis. The best UK evidence in support of this position was gathered in the Psychiatric Morbidity Survey. This research was carried out in the early 1990s, with over 11,000 participants in four separate surveys (Bebbington *et al.*, 1998; Jenkins *et al.*, 1997; Mason and Wilkinson, 1996; Jenkins and Meltzer, 1995; Meltzer *et al.*, 1995). It distinguished between neurotic disorders (mixed anxiety and depressive disorder, generalised anxiety disorder, depressive episode, phobias, obsessive compulsive disorder and panic disorder) and non-neurotic disorders (functional psychoses, alcohol dependence and drug dependence). Women showed higher one-year prevalence rates for all the neurotic disorders, similar rates for the functional psychoses and much lower rates for alcohol and drug dependence, when compared with men. Within the neurotic disorders, the difference between men and women was greatest for the most common category – mixed anxiety and depressive disorder – calculated as 99 cases per 1,000 for women and 54 cases per 1,000 for men in the week prior to the survey (Meltzer *et al.*, 1995). This two-to-one gender differential in anxiety disorders was also confirmed in the American NCS, with women having a one-year prevalence of 23 per cent, while for men it was 12 per cent (Kessler *et al.*, 1994: 12).

Some indirect, international comparisons lend further support to these findings, as reflected in the work of Regier and his colleagues, who also presented the American ECA study findings in the context of material from other parts of the world (Regier *et al.*, 1993). Based on data from a range of European countries as well as Australia and Uganda, Regier *et al.* (1993) examined studies in which the participants were asked to indicate any symptoms they had experienced in the month prior to the interview. Although highlighting the difficulties involved in making such international comparisons, particularly in light of the wide variation in prevalence rates across nations, they reported a significant gender imbalance in relation to affective disorders and anxiety disorders. In other words, although there were some slight differences between men and women across countries in terms of the specific symptoms reported, overall monthly prevalence rates for affective disorders (including depression) and anxiety disorders were much higher among women than among men. As Regier *et al.*, in summarising their findings, conclude:

> Affective disorders were found in women at about twice the rate as in men for London, Australia and Athens. Anxiety disorders were much more variable in their sex ratio, with rates four times higher for women than men in London and Athens, but a somewhat higher male rate in Australia. (Regier *et al.*, 1993: 984)

The vulnerability of women to anxiety and depression has elicited extensive research activity throughout the western world (Zlotnick *et al.*, 1996; Zerbe, 1995; Bebbington *et al.*, 1991; Pilowsky *et al.*, 1991). One interesting study is that of Walters (1993), who sought to clarify how Canadian women viewed their own health and illness. The 356 women, who participated in the study, reported very high levels of stress (60 per cent), of anxiety (44 per cent) and of depression (35 per cent). These were not surprising findings in themselves. What was new was the women's interpretation of the experience of these symptoms and their perception of the causes. As expected, they spoke of multiple demands from family and work, of 'overload', with no time to rest, and of isolation or lack of a confidante. However, what was unusual was the fact that they recounted these demands in a way that did not dwell on personal culpability but rather on the inevitable impact of the social situation (work and family) in which they found themselves:

> Gendered caring roles, family structure, women's position in the labour market and their financial resources intertwined and threatened women's mental health. While private issues were not consistently discussed in public and political terms, they were often located in this context. (Walters, 1993: 401)

These women did not medicalise their own condition as is sometimes suggested. Most of them defined their anxieties and stress as normal reactions to everyday life. They did not conceptualise them as illness, although they did admit that they could be potential risk factors for physical illness. These modern Canadian women were describing the same process as that described by Edward Shorter (1990) in a study of hysteria in nineteenth-century Austria. Women selected the medical route to help only when all other avenues for dealing with an overwhelming social burden were closed. This is not to deny, however, the well-established fact that a higher proportion of women than men seek medical help for mental health problems and are, therefore, more likely than men to receive a psychiatric diagnosis (Busfield, 1999, 1996, 1994; Ussher, 1991). However, whether or not this is due to the fact that women have a more difficult life than men, or that they are more likely than men to have their problems labelled as mental illness, is open to debate (for further discussion, see Chapter 8).

The mental health of men

The low visibility of men in official psychiatric statistics has led, in the past, to the false conclusion that men have better mental health than women. The statistics that are available are difficult to interpret because some of the mental health problems most commonly associated with men – those related to alcohol or drug dependence, those associated with suicide, and those labelled personality disorder – have, until very recently, often not featured in psychiatric statistics. The absence of these conditions from these statistics may be explained by the fact that these specific problems were not regarded as amenable to psychiatric treatment and were, therefore, marginalised within the mental health care system. However, men are clearly visible when common mental illnesses – such as depression, anxiety or neurosis – are examined, as these are recognised as treatable by psychiatry.

What is interesting, from a gender perspective, is that although men suffer from a range of recognised psychiatric symptoms – anxiety, depression, phobias and panic attacks – they have a lower prevalence rate than women for all of these symptoms, though the difference is greater for some than for others. The National Psychiatric Morbidity Survey – carried out in England, Wales and Scotland in 1993 and 1994 – found that 'all disorders, except psychosis and drug and alcohol dependence were commoner in women than men' (Jenkins *et al.*, 1997: 783). When participants in this survey were asked about symptoms experienced in the week prior to the interview, almost 20 per cent of men reported fatigue, sleep problems, irritability, and worry – all symptoms of neurosis. Almost 10 per cent of men reported depression and anxiety, while between 3 and 5 per cent reported obsessions, phobias, and lost concentration (Jenkins *et al.*, 1997: 781). In other words, depression and anxiety are major mental health problems for men, affecting approximately one out of every 10 individuals. This statistic is confirmed by American research that suggests a yearly prevalence of around 10 per cent for depression and 12 per cent for anxiety among men (Kessler *et al.*, 1994).

However, all of these men do not necessarily seek help from the mental health care system. Many of them show up instead in the suicide statistics – a major area of concern in today's society. It appears that the rate of suicide is increasing among men in the

UK as it is in many other countries in the western world (for discussion, see Kaplan and Sadock, 1995). According to O'Dowd and Jewell (1998: 51), there were 2,787 deaths from suicide among men and 783 among women in England and Wales in 1995. They suggest that the numbers in themselves are less worrying than the trends. It appears that, since 1975, the rate has been increasing among men and decreasing among women, and that this trend is clearest among 15–29 year olds in disadvantaged areas.

Suicide is often linked to depression but, as rates of depression are higher in women and suicide rates lower, there are still questions to be answered as to why men commit suicide rather than seek help for depressive symptoms. The general consensus of opinion is that the unwillingness among men to look for help is linked to notions of masculinity and unwillingness to appear weak or afraid. Joseph Pleck (1981), an American psychologist, was one of the first clinicians to suggest that the male role might be oppressive for men and that conformity to it might be psychologically damaging. However, his viewpoint was not highly regarded within psychiatry and it is only recently that there is an interest in exploring the links between the burdens of the male role and behaviour that places the health of men at risk.

This risky behaviour includes alcohol and drug abuse. However, as briefly mentioned earlier, it is only in recent years that statistics on alcohol and drug dependence have been defined as indicators of mental disorder – a statistic in which men (particularly young men) feature prominently. The American Epidemiologic Catchment Area (ECA) Survey, for example, was one of the first empirical studies to acknowledge substance dependence and personality disorder as mental conditions in need of professional attention in the same way as depression or anxiety disorders (Robins and Regier, 1991). This was followed by the National Co-Morbidity Survey (NCS) – a study specifically aimed at exploring the relationship between substance dependence and recognised mental illnesses. The NCS found men twice as likely as women to have a substance dependence problem – with a lifetime prevalence of almost 36 per cent for men and 18 per cent for women (Kessler *et al.*, 1994: 12). In other words, over one-third of the male population in the USA are estimated to be dependent on alcohol or drugs at some stage in their lives.

A further examination of the figures showed that alcohol dependence was a more widespread health problem than drug dependence, being second only to depression in the overall figures on mental disorders among men. One in five men reported having been dependent on alcohol at some time in their lives (lifetime prevalence of 20 per cent) and more than one in ten had been dependent in the previous year (one-year prevalence of 11 per cent). In contrast, one in every 12 women reported having been dependent on alcohol at some time in their lives (lifetime prevalence of 8.2 per cent) while one in 27 had been dependent in the previous year (one-year prevalence of 3.7 per cent). The ECA study reported similar trends, with a slightly higher lifetime prevalence level for men (Robins and Regier, 1991: 88, Table 5.3). Both studies found that younger men had much higher rates of alcohol and drug dependence than older men. For example, the NCS found that those aged 25–34 years were twice as likely as those aged 45–54 years to report substance dependency (Kessler *et al.*, 1994: 15).

Similar patterns are found in the UK. In the Psychiatric Morbidity Survey, for example, men were three times more likely than women to be alcohol dependent and twice as likely to be drug dependent. In addition, men aged 20–24 years were found to be at particular risk, with a one-year prevalence of 18 per cent for alcohol dependence and 11 per cent for drug dependence (Meltzer *et al.*, 1995: 68; see also, Jenkins *et al.*, 1997). Other statistical evidence from the Office for National Statistics (ONS) indicates that overall alcohol consumption in the population in the UK increased in the period between 1950 and 1990, but it has levelled off since then (Charlton and Murphy, 1997a: 116). However, alcohol-related mortality continues to increase among men though not among women. The situation in relation to drug dependence is much more serious – both drug dependence and drug-related mortality have increased significantly since the 1970s, with men affected much more than women (Charlton and Murphy, 1997a: 127). Clearly, the mental health problems associated with alcohol and drug dependence have to be recognised and tackled within the mainstream mental health service. Otherwise, an increasing number of men will be excluded from receiving help and treatment for their mental health problems.

A similar omission – in terms of mainstream mental health service recognition and provision – also arises when personality disorders are considered. This is the other major area of controversy in relation to the visibility of men in psychiatric statistics – the debate on what is called 'anti-social personality disorder' in the USA, and 'personality disorder' in the UK. This condition, largely regarded as untreatable by psychiatrists, is often omitted from statistics on mental disorder. However, according to Robins and Regier (1991: 258), anti-social personality disorder, which they define as 'the violation of the rights of others and a general lack of conformity to social norms', constitutes a mental disorder and should, therefore, be included in mental health statistics. More specifically, the reason for its inclusion, according to these two highly regarded researchers in the ECA study in the USA, is that it meets all the criteria of a mental disorder in that 'its symptoms are highly inter-correlated, making it a coherent syndrome . . . it has a genetic component . . . and it occurs in and is recognized by every society, no matter what its economic system' (Robins and Regier, 1991: 258)

It could be argued, however, that to include this category is simply to medicalise criminal behaviour. Robins and Regier, as they were aware of this criticism, specifically tested for an association between a criminal history and the diagnosis of anti-social personality disorder but found a general lack of support for this position. For their analysis, again based on the ECA study in the USA, they used the definition of this disorder from the American classification system for mental illnesses – the Diagnostic Statistical Manual, Revised Version Three (DSM-III). As illustrated by the quotation below, they were surprised to find little empirical support for a direct link between a criminal record and the presence of an anti-social personality disorder in the individuals being studied. In other words, the correlation between the two variables was not significantly high in this instance. As the researchers, in summarising their findings, conclude:

In fact less than half (47 per cent) of those positive for the DSM-III diagnosis have a significant record of arrest (defined as two or more arrests other than for a moving traffic violation or any felony conviction). Rather than criminality, the adult symptoms that typify the anti-social personality are job troubles (found in 94 per cent), violence (found in 85 per cent), multiple moving traffic offences (found in 72 per cent), and severe marital difficulties (desertion, multiple separations or divorces, multiple infidelities), found in 67 per cent. (Robins and Regier, 1991: 260)

When the extent of this disorder within the total population was examined, however, as expected, only a minority of individuals could be diagnosed in terms of this condition. For example, not only did Robins and Regier report a lifetime prevalence of just 2.6 per cent within the USA population as a whole, but less than half of these people had experienced active symptoms in the previous year (one-year prevalence of 1.2 per cent). As would be expected, however, men had a higher lifetime (4.5 per cent) and one-year (2.1 per cent) prevalence of a personality disorder than women (lifetime prevalence of 0.8 per cent and one-year prevalence of 0.4 per cent). As with crime statistics, young men were found to be more prone to this condition than older men, a finding that was consistent across ethnic boundaries. In the UK, because of the controversy surrounding the diagnosis of personality disorder, it is impossible to get comparable statistics, but it is likely that similar gender and crime patterns prevail.

To summarise this section on the mental health problems of men, it is clear that although a small number of men express their distress in ways that can be recognised as symptoms of depression or anxiety, many do not. Rather, they either engage in high-risk behaviour – such as alcohol or drug abuse – or they commit suicide. Because of this, many men with mental health problems either never come to the attention of the health care system, or they are labelled as untreatable within that system.

Gender and the use of services

Although it has been accepted generally that there are gender differences in almost all psychiatric statistics, it is surprising how few studies on the use of services include gender as a variable. Fortunately, recent research has begun to address the issue in a systematic way. From the available evidence, it is clear that a number of patterns are emerging, though some of them are not consistent with each other. Based on the arguments presented previously, we suggest that if substance dependence and personality disorders are included in the definition of mental disorder some interesting conclusions can be drawn, that are quite different from those if these conditions are excluded. The evidence in support of this position is as follows.

First, as shown in the American studies, if substance dependence and personality disorders are included in definitions of mental disorder, women and men may be considered to be at an equal risk of having a current mental disorder – with a 20 per cent one-year prevalence. In other words, one out of five men and one out of five women would expect to experience some mental health problem in any given year. Second, men would be considered to be at a higher risk of developing a mental disorder in their lifetime – 36 per cent lifetime prevalence for men and 30 per cent for women (Robins and Regier, 1991). In other words, just over one-third of men and just under one-third of women would expect to have mental health problems in their lifetime.

From these findings, it could be inferred that women and men have almost the same level of need for mental health care at any given time – with men having a slightly higher level of need than women over a longer time period. Mental health services, therefore, need to be flexible and varied to cater for the very different ways in which men and women manifest their mental health problems. However, it appears that this is not the case. Throughout Europe and the USA, mental health services tend to cater for women rather than men – probably due to the fact that women are substantially higher users of these services than men, just as they are higher users of general health services (see Chapter 4). Furthermore, this seems to be particularly the case when primary care, or community-based services, are considered.

Focusing initially on primary care services, existing research confirms that women predominate in statistics on the use of medication and other primary care services for mental health problems. They are prescribed approximately twice as many psychotropic drugs per head as men throughout Europe and North America (for a review of the studies, see Ashton, 1991). For example in a study of 133,081 patients of general practitioners in the UK in the early 1970s, the prescription rate was 20 per cent for women and 10 per cent for men, with the prescription rates rising with age, but maintaining the same gender pattern. In a study of 24,633 similar patients in Boston (USA) during the same era, the findings were even more startling, with 25 per cent of women and 15 per cent of men receiving psychotropic drugs. A cross-national study in 1980–81 of sedative use, which is the most commonly prescribed of this group of drugs, confirmed the general pattern. In all of the countries, the female-to-male ratio was approximately 2 to 1. The highest ratio was reported in Belgium – 21 per cent for women and 13 per cent for men, and the lowest in the Netherlands – 9 per cent for women and 6 per cent for men (for all of these statistics, see Ashton, 1991: 31).

Explanations for the differential prescription rates for men and women are conjectural to a large extent, as there are few studies to analyse the prescription decisions by doctors. Research evidence that does exist, however, suggests three inter-related factors in explaining this phenomenon. First, male doctors are more likely to perceive a physical illness as a psychological one when the patient is a woman. Second, medical advertising reinforces this perception of women being prone to mental health problems. For example, women appear more often in advertisements for psychoactive drugs, in contrast to non-psychoactive drugs where men appear more often. Third, because of both the above factors, this type of medication is more socially acceptable for women than for men (for discussion, see Ashton, 1991). All of these explanations support the feminist arguments on the particular social construction of 'mental illness behaviour', which makes the discourse of mental illness and medical treatment an acceptable vehicle for women but not for men (Shorter, 1990; Showalter, 1987).

The low level of use by men of primary care services for mental health problems fits into a pattern of low levels of service use by men in relation to other health problems (Conrad, 1997: 52, 496; Doyal, 1995). Men are reluctant help-seekers in relation to both physical and mental health. This pattern is confirmed in the American ECA study, which had, as one of its main research purposes, the estimation of the level of unmet mental health need in the general population. In order to establish this need, those judged to have active symptoms of a psychiatric disorder were asked if they had sought or received help. The answers were startling in terms of specific groups in the population. For example, many differences were found in relation to gender, education and race. Only 19 per cent of the people, who reported having active psychiatric symptoms, had received any form of treatment – 2.4 per cent had received in-patient treatment in the previous year and 16.4 per cent received out-patient treatment in the previous six months (Robins and Regier, 1991: 341, Table 13.5). Women received more treatment than men – 23 per cent as against 14 per cent – and men and women with a high-school education were slightly more likely to receive treatment than those who had not. Married men without a high-school education were the least likely to use services. According to these findings, most people at least three out of four women and six out of seven men – with mental health problems do not receive medical treatment at all.

In an in-depth analysis of what happened to those who did seek and receive treatment, Shapiro et al. (1984) found that there were two major gender differences. In each survey area, more women than men made mental health visits to their health care provider, but the men were more likely to be seen by a mental health specialist than were the women. Studies on referrals to specialist psychiatric services in Europe found a similar pattern in the filtering of people from general primary care services to specialist mental health services either in the community or in hospital. In comparison with women, fewer men are diagnosed as having a mental illness, but a larger proportion of those diagnosed are referred for specialist assessment and treatment (see Verhaak, 1993; Wilkinson, 1989). This means that they are judged to be more seriously ill and are, therefore, more likely to receive more intensive treatment, which often involves institution-based care.

The gender pattern in the use of institution-based mental health treatment has been the subject of the most important sociological debates on the relationship between gender and mental health. As already indicated in the introduction to this chapter, when treatment was concentrated in publicly-funded mental hospitals from the eighteenth century to the mid-twentieth century, women were in the majority in the in-patient population (Busfield, 1999; Showalter, 1987). However, as indicated already, there were exceptions to this rule – one of the most notable being the Republic of Ireland where men have always outnumbered women in mental health beds (Cleary, 1997; Prior, 1993; Finnane, 1981).

Since the 1960s, when the movement to de-institutionalise people from large mental hospitals began, the patterns of both service delivery and service use have changed throughout the western world. Community mental health services have expanded, publicly-funded hospital beds have decreased, and independently-run (commercial and non-profit) hospitals and residential facilities have increased. Current research indicates that, in the USA, the proportion of men in institution-based treatment is increasing. However, men are most likely to be admitted to facilities catering specifically for substance dependence and to involuntary (compulsory) hospital treatment (for discussion, see Watkins and Callicutt, 1997). In the UK, the existing evidence suggests that women continue to be higher users of institution-based care than do men. However, some researchers, such as Sarah Payne (1995, 1996), have found evidence of an upward trend in admission rates among younger men. Others, such as Lelliot *et al.* (1994), found that young men (aged 18–34 years) predominate among new long-stay patients in England and Wales. However, because of the high numbers of older women in the patient population as a whole, this fact is often overlooked.

Sociological perspectives on gender differences

What may explain these changing differences in mental health statistics and health service use between men and women? Current sociological debate offers two competing theoretical explanations to account for these gender-specific changes, or the increasing visibility of men in statistics on psychiatric morbidity and the use of mental health care services. These two competing theoretical explanations are known in the literature as the social causation versus the social construction perspective.

Box 7.1 Sociological explanations for gender differences in mental health

- Social causation approach
- Social construction approach

Focusing initially on the social causation approach, advocates of this position suggest that these gender-specific changes may be attributed to a real increase in mental problems among men and a decrease among women. In other words, they argue that men are mentally less healthy and women are mentally more healthy than previously. According to social causation theorists, it is this factor – gender-specific changes in the actual experience of mental illness – which accounts for the increasing visibility of men in statistics on psychiatric morbidity and mental health service use. Researchers, working from this perspective, focus on the impact of modern life as experienced by men, most notably in terms of the increasing demands of an oppressive and stereotypically-based male role, to account for differences in mental health patterns between men and women (see Pleck, 1981; David and Brannon, 1976).

Proponents of the social constructionist perspective, however, reject this view. In direct contrast to social causation theorists, they argue that these gender-specific changes in patterns of mental health service use have little to do with changes in the experience of mental health problems. Rather, according to this perspective, it is the re-conceptualisation of mental disorder from a stereotypical female focus to an equally stereotypical male focus – and not changes in the actual experience of mental health problems – that accounts for the increasing visibility of men in mental health statistics. In other words, it is this factor – the inclusion of a range of previously excluded male problems, such as alcohol and drug dependency and, also, personality disorders – which now leaves men more vulnerable to a diagnosis of mental disorder and to institution-based treatment.

In summary, then, there are two competing perspectives to account for these gender-specific changes in mental health statistics. While these two perspectives offer different explanations to account for these changes, both agree on the increasing visibility of men in statistics on psychiatric morbidity and health service use (for further discussion, see Chapters 8 and 9). It is with this finding in mind – the suggested increase in the visibility of men in mental health statistics – that the following discussion focuses on gender differences in service use in relation to institution-based mental health care in the UK.

The use of secondary care services – men replacing women

As we have seen earlier, it may be said that, in general, women admit to higher levels of mental illness and make greater use of both primary and secondary health care services than do men. Traditionally, men have been extremely reluctant help-seekers in relation to both physical and mental health. More recent research in the USA and elsewhere, however, suggests that this may no longer be the case where mental health is concerned. For example, not only are men becoming increasingly visible in statistics on psychiatric morbidity, but this seems to be particularly the case when alcohol and drug dependency are considered (Meltzer *et al.*, 1995; Robins and Regier, 1991). To what extent, however, are these increasing levels of reported psychiatric symptoms among men beginning to translate into their greater use of secondary care services within the mental health care system in the UK?

The data already presented in Chapter 3 provided some indirect evidence in support of this proposition. This evidence is based on a comparison of the populations using institution-based services for physical and mental health (see Table 3.2 and associated discussion). As shown there, the analysis of census data suggests that while only a minority of both the male and female populations using these services are concentrated in mental health facilities, the proportionate presence in mental health beds is higher for men than for women. For example, in 1991, of the total male population in institution-based care in the UK, 15 per cent were in mental health facilities, while of the total female population in similar care, only 7 per cent were in mental health facilities. The question arises, therefore, 'Will this finding hold when a more direct examination of these populations is undertaken?'. In other words, when men and women are compared directly, are men now becoming greater users of institution-based mental health services than are women?

Table 7.1 provides the answer to this question by calculating the proportion of men and women in the population in institution-based mental health care. This population includes those in all hospitals and residential facilities (health and social care) designated for mental health care. The data includes all sectors of pro-

Table 7.1 Gender differences in levels of bed occupancy in mental health facilities in the UK, 1921–91

Year	Men (%)	Women (%)	Gender gap (%)	Number of occupants
1921/26	45.3	54.7	−9	139,597
1931/37	46.3	53.7	−7	181,632
1951	45.9	54.1	−8	223,250
1971	47.6	52.4	−5	199,059
1981	48.6	51.4	−3	135,691
1991	50.0	50.0	0	52,379

Note: Because of the absence of distinguishing data between physical and mental health facilities in Northern Ireland, a UK figure could not be calculated for the 1961 census period.

Source: England & Wales and Scotland Census, 1921, 1931, 1951, 1971, 1981, 1991; Northern Ireland Census, 1926, 1937, 1951, 1971, 1981, 1991.

vision – public, commercial and non-profit. However, facilities for people with learning disability are excluded from the analysis, because the issues in relation to the use of services are completely different. Similar to previous examinations of the secondary care sector, this information is derived from an analysis of UK census data on occupants of all designated mental health beds in all but one decade – 1961 – since the 1920s. Because of the absence of distinguishing data between physical and mental health facilities in Northern Ireland in 1961, a UK figure could not be calculated for this census period. The questions being asked in this investigation are as follows:

(1) Are there gender differences in the use of institution-based mental health care?
(2) Is there any indication that the gender pattern in the use of these services is changing?

If we look at Table 7.1, we find the answer to our first question. Throughout most of the twentieth century, there were substantial gender differences in the use of residential mental health services. Women featured more prominently than men up until 1991, at which time men and women became equal users of these services. A closer look at the information, presented as a gender gap, or the percentage difference between men and women, shows that this gap – with women predominating – was greatest at the beginning of the century (a gap of 9 per cent). This pattern held in the first half of the century. As men increased in this population in the second half of the century, the gap decreased until it finally disappeared in 1991.

This absence of a gender gap in the use of residential mental health services in the UK must be considered an extremely important finding for two reasons. First, contrary to traditionally-held notions of women as the 'madder sex', the results of this investigation suggest that, at least as far as secondary care services are concerned, men and women are now equally likely to use these services. Second, and more importantly, however, it further confirms existing international research on the increasing visibility of men in statistics on psychiatric morbidity and on mental health service usage. In other words, gender trends in the UK are now showing some of the same characteristics as those emerging in other national and international research – the increasing visibility of men in institution-based mental health care (Watkins and Callicutt, 1997; Payne, 1996, 1995; Lelliot *et al.*, 1994). It may no longer be said, therefore, that women in the UK are higher users of mental health services than men. They are now equal users of this very large section of mental health services – institution-based care.

The second clear pattern shown in Table 7.1 is that this disproportionate increase in men in the population in UK mental health facilities coincided with a decrease in the actual size of this population, caused by the de-institutionalisation movement in the second half of the twentieth century. The total population in mental health beds plummeted from a high of 223,250 in 1951 to less than a quarter of this size in 1991 – to 52,379 people. In other words, as bed numbers decreased in the mental health sector in the UK, it appears that clinicians were making highly gendered judgements as to the use of this scarce resource. The fact that the judgements were gendered was not surprising in itself. It had happened for years, resulting in a tendency to admit more women than men to institution-based care. What was new, however, was that the judgement now 'favoured' men over women, resulting in a tendency to admit many more men to hospitals and care facilities than in the past (for further discussion, see Chapters 8 and 9).

Is this also the case, however, when the three constituent parts of the UK – England and Wales, Scotland and Northern Ireland – are investigated separately? In other words, are men and women now equal in terms of their use of institution-based care in all three regions of the UK? It is with this question in mind that the final section of this chapter focuses on both gender and regional differences in the use of secondary care services within the mental health care system in the UK.

Gender differences in service use – the importance of region

The data in Table 7.2 show us regional differences in the gender balance in the population in mental health facilities in the UK during the last three decades of the twentieth century. To allow a distinction between the various regions, the table is divided into three panels. Panel A, which presents the results for England and Wales, Panel B, which shows the equivalent data for Scotland, and Panel C, which shows the equivalent information for Northern Ireland. The results suggest that, while men are now dominant over women in terms of their use of these facilities in England and Wales, it is women, and not men, who continue to predominate in both Scotland and Northern Ireland. Furthermore, this is particularly and increasingly the case in Scotland, where the gender gap in the use of these services, or the difference in the proportion between women and men, has actually widened since 1981.

Focusing initially on England and Wales, which has the largest population in mental health facilities, the results suggest a clear change in the gender composition of this population (see Table 7.2, Panel A). The gender balance has reversed – from a dominance of women over men in the early 1970s, to a dominance of men over women in the early 1990s (for further discussion, see Chapter 8; and Prior and Hayes, 2001b). In 1991, 52 per cent of the population in institution-based mental health care in

Table 7.2 Gender differences in levels of bed occupancy in mental health facilities in the UK by region, 1971–91

	Men (%)	Women (%)	Gender gap (%)	Number of occupants
Panel A: England & Wales				
1971	47.4	52.6	−5	169,190
1981	48.8	51.2	−2	113,687
1991	51.8	48.2	+4	38,963
Panel B: Scotland				
1971	48.7	51.3	−3	24,925
1981	47.9	52.1	−4	18,850
1991	43.1	56.9	−14	10,079
Panel C: Northern Ireland				
1971	49.7	50.3	−1	4,944
1981	46.7	53.3	−7	3,154
1991	48.7	51.3	−3	3,337

Source: England & Wales, Scotland, and Northern Ireland Census, 1971, 1981 and 1991.

England and Wales were men as compared to 48 per cent for women. Thus, at least as far as this particular region is concerned, the gender composition of the population in mental health facilities is now following the pattern already established in the USA – the higher and disproportionate use by men of this type of care and treatment (Watkins and Callicutt, 1997; Sanguineti *et al.*, 1996).

This is not the case, however, in either Scotland or Northern Ireland (see Table 7.2, Panel B and Panel C, respectively). In both these regions, the gender gap – with women predominating – remains, though to a much lesser degree in Northern Ireland than in Scotland. In fact, since 1981, whereas the gender gap decreased by four per cent in Northern Ireland from 7 per cent to 3 per cent, it further increased in Scotland, rising from just 4 per cent in 1981 to 14 per cent in 1991. In other words, although women continue to be higher users of institution-based mental health care than men in both these regions, this is particularly and increasingly the case in Scotland.

It is interesting to note, however, that at least as far as Scotland is concerned, this increase in the use of institution-based mental health care by women coincided with a dramatic numerical drop in the cared-for population. In line with de-institutionalisation policies throughout the UK, the number of people in mental health facilities more than halved between 1971 and 1991 in Scotland – from 24,925 to 10,079. Thus, during this time period, more men than women were discharged from mental health beds, leaving a much higher proportion of women than of men in these facilities. Northern Ireland, in contrast, saw a marginal increase in its population in institution-based care between 1981 and 1991 – from 3,154 to 3,337 (for further discussion on Northern Ireland, see Chapter 9; and Prior and Hayes, 2001a).

In conclusion, then, international research evidence points to the need for an analysis of the experience of mental health problems and the use of mental health services in gender terms. This evidence tells us that women more often seek help for mental disorder but are often prescribed drugs by their general practitioner and not referred to specialist psychiatric services. Men, on the other hand, find it difficult to seek help and are often seriously ill before they come to the notice of the medical services (Verhaak, 1993; Robins and Regier, 1991). Having accessed the services, women are more likely to use community services successfully and to recover from severe mental disorders (Pfeiffer *et al.*, 1996). On the other hand, men who access the mental health system are more likely to become heavy users of psychiatric services and to appear in the new long-stay hospital populations (Kent *et al.*, 1995b; Lelliot *et al.*, 1994). Finally, gender trends in diagnosis and treatment are changing. It may no longer be claimed that women outnumber men in all mental health statistics. Men are becoming increasingly visible in statistics on psychiatric morbidity, on the use of services for substance dependence and on hospital in-patient treatment (Prior and Hayes, 2001b; Sanguineti *et al.*, 1996; Robins and Regier, 1991).

In the next two chapters, we will explore two of the stereotypical notions that still prevail in the public imagination – that women are 'madder' than men and that young men prefer to be labelled 'bad' rather than 'mad'. Both notions derive from the fact that women have been more visible than men in psychiatric statistics. Through this exploration, we hope not only to challenge public opinion on the experience of mental health problems but also to call into question the assumptions that underpin many mental health care systems in western society today.

Summary

- Women have a much higher visibility in psychiatric statistics than have men
- Over one in five women and about one in ten men claim to have experienced either depression or anxiety at some time in their lives
- Men are twice as likely as women to report substance dependency – alcohol or drugs
- Although women predominated in the population in institution-based care in the UK for most of the twentieth century, since the 1990s, women and men have because equal users of these services
- Different gender patterns in the use of mental health services are evident within the UK and require further research

8 Women as the 'Madder' Sex

Introduction

Until recently, it was widely believed that women were more prone to mental illness than men, as indicated by their higher visibility in most statistics on mental illness. This numerical predominance of women in psychiatric statistics confirmed stereotypical notions of women as 'mad', and led to extensive debates on the reasons for the greater vulnerability of women both to the experience of mental health problems and to treatment in a psychiatric setting (for discussion, see Chapter 7). In recent years, however, this belief has been increasingly challenged. This is particularly the case in the USA, where a number of empirical studies have found a notable increase not only in the number of men reporting psychiatric symptoms but also in terms of their use of institution-based mental health care. Examples of these empirical studies, which have been discussed in earlier chapters, include the ECA and the NCS, in which men reported higher levels of mental disorder over their lifetimes than did women (Kessler *et al.*, 1994; Robins and Regier, 1991). Studies on institution-based care, particularly those examining statistics on involuntary (compulsory) admissions, have also found this pattern. For example, men formed the majority (58 per cent) of the 2,200 patients admitted on an involuntary basis to hospitals in Philadelphia in the early 1990s (Sanguineti *et al.*, 1996).

A similar pattern – the increasing presence of men in reported psychiatric morbidity and in mental health service use – is also beginning to emerge in the UK, as evidenced in the work of Bebbington *et al.* (1994), Flannigan *et al.* (1994a, 1994b), Lelliot *et al.* (1994) and Thomas *et al.* (1993). Lelliot and colleagues carried out a study of all new long-stay (NLS) patients in mental health facilities in England and Wales. They found, for example, that not only had the proportion of men in this population increased substantially since 1972 – when it stood at 48 per cent – but that, by 1992, men constituted a clear majority (57 per cent). Furthermore, the vast majority of young NLS patients in these facilities were single males, aged 18–34 years. The other studies were on a much smaller scale but showed increases in psychiatric admissions among younger men in London (Bebbington *et al.*, 1994; Flannigan *et al.*, 1994a, 1994b) and in Manchester (Thomas *et al.*, 1993). However, because of the higher numbers of older women among overall admissions in these cities, this increase did not show up as a change in the overall gender balance. Payne (1995, 1996) found a similar pattern in her study of psychiatric admission rates for England and Wales during the 1980s. Although overall admissions were still dominated by women, the trend was different in the younger age group (18–25 years), where the admission rates for men were catching up with, and sometimes surpassing those for women.

As discussed briefly in Chapter 7, two competing theoretical explanations – the social causation versus the social construction perspective – have been proposed to account for these gender-specific changes, or the increasing visibility of men in mental health statistics. Here we present a more detailed discussion of these two perspectives as a basis for understanding the case studies that follow in this and in the next chapter.

Social causation explanation

The social causation perspective, as previously explained, suggests that these gender-specific changes result from a real increase in mental health problems among men and a decrease among women. Studies based within this theoretical framework seek links between the mental health of men and changes in modern life as a whole. For example, Joseph Pleck, a psychologist writing in the late 1970s and early 1980s, took up the challenge of feminists who argued that a patriarchal society damaged the health of women. He suggested that it was also damaging for men, many of whom were oppressed by the male role (Pleck, 1981).

David and Brannon (1976) had already described the stereotypical male role in terms of four dimensions. The first – *no sissy stuff* – is the need for men to be different from women. The second – *the big wheel* – is the need to be superior to others. The third dimension – *the sturdy oak* – is the need to be independent and self-reliant. The fourth, or final, dimension – *give 'em Hell* – is the need to be more powerful than others, through violence if necessary. Although not everyone agrees with this stereotypical characterisation of the male role, previous research suggests that some elements may ring true. There is something, for example, about the male role that encourages some men, at least, to lead their lives in a way that contributes to their higher rates of mortality and consequent shorter life expectancy than women (Courtenay, 2000; Kimmell and Messner, 1995). In fact, some of these writers go so far as to suggest that this role has become more oppressive than previously – a trend that would explain the increase in mental health problems among men (Edley and Wetherell, 1995). Others, however, disagree, suggesting instead that it is the increased recognition of the possible negative impact of the male role on health that has led to the higher visibility of men in mental health statistics (see Gomez, 1993).

In a similar vein, Payne (1995, 1996), also writing from this theoretical perspective, identified a number of new and additional factors in the lives of some men – particularly young men in disadvantaged areas – that might be linked to increases in reported mental illness among men. She suggests that redundancy, not only from employment but also from a meaningful male role in the family, has had an impact on how society views young men. They are increasingly seen as disconnected from the normal channels of social control – the economy and the family – and, therefore, are in need of more public control. Payne related changes in both psychiatric and penal discourse, on both men and women, to changes in patterns of employment and of family life. The young men most at risk of hospitalisation and of imprisonment were most likely to be unemployed and single:

> Thus, as young men have become more detached from the world of paid work, and from family and paternal responsibilities, they have become more visible in their discontent, and at the same time, the need for control of this group has increased and become more visible. (Payne, 1996: 174)

Other evidence of increasing stress in the lives of men comes from the 'self help' literature now emerging in relation to men's health (see Luck *et al.*, 2000) and from general sociological and psychological literature on masculinity (see Courtenay, 2000; Edley and Wetherell, 1995; Connell, 1995; Gomez, 1993). All of this work highlights a crisis in the male identity brought about by changes in the role of women in society – changes that have impacted substantially on the lives of men at work and in the home. Of course, the fact that men have more stress in their lives does not necessarily lead them to seek help in the health system – it is more likely that they will show their distress by turning to alcohol or drugs or, as a last resort, to suicide. Courtenay (2000), for example, who writes extensively on the interaction between the masculine role and health behaviour among American men, describes this reluctance in the following way:

> Indeed, in response to depression, men are more likely than women to rely on themselves, to withdraw socially, to try to talk themselves out of depression or to convince themselves that depression is 'stupid'. Nearly half of men over age 49 nationally who reported experiencing an extended depression did not discuss it with anyone. Instead, men tend to engage in private activities, including drinking and drug use, designed to distract themselves or to alleviate their depression. Denial of depression is one of the means men use to demonstrate

masculinities and to avoid assignment to a lower-status position relative to women and other men. (Courtenay, 2000: 1397)

Social constructionist explanation

The second, or alternative sociological perspective, used to account for gender-specific changes in mental health statistics, is the social constructionist explanation. As discussed earlier, advocates of this position totally reject the social causation explanation. They argue that gender-specific changes in patterns of reported psychiatric morbidity and mental health service use have little to do with changes in the experience of mental health problems. Rather, according to this perspective, it is the re-conceptualisation of mental disorder from a female focus to a male focus – and not changes in the actual experience of mental problems – that accounts for the increasing visibility of men in mental health statistics. In other words, it is this specific factor – the growing inclusion of stereotypical notions about male behaviour in the discourse of mental disorder – that explains the increasing and disproportionate vulnerability of men to a diagnosis of mental disorder and to institution-based treatment.

The arguments are as follows. Past conceptualisations of mental disorder identified women, rather than men, as the group most susceptible to mental health problems requiring psychiatric treatment. Categories of mental illness were almost exclusively operationalised in terms that matched traditional stereotypical notions of female problems – for example, depression and anxiety. In contrast, conditions commonly associated with men – personality disorder and substance dependence – were excluded from these categories. In the past, this translated into a range of professional decisions to over-diagnose and over-treat women (for discussion, see Loring and Powell, 1988). However, this is no longer the case.

In recent years, they suggest, there has been a gradual change in the conceptualisation of mental disorder in the western world. Past definitions, for example, based on behaviour associated with hysteria, anxiety and depression are now giving way to notions of dangerousness or risk to the public, characteristics more often associated with men than with women. In other words, stereo-typical notions about male behaviour, such as a perceived greater potential for violence towards self and society, have now become part of the discourse of mental disorder. This is most apparent in the USA, but is also evident in debates surrounding recent changes in mental health law in a number of European coun-tries, including the UK (see Manning and Shaw, 1999). Social constructionists suggest that it is this factor – the inclusion of stereotypical notions of male behaviour in the conceptualisation of mental disorder – that may explain recent gender trends in mental health statistics. These trends are a growing visibility of men in measures of psychiatric morbidity, and indications of an increasing susceptibility among men to institutionalisation in the mental health systems of the western world (for discussion, see Miller, 1993; La Fond and Durham, 1992). They also suggest that it has led to a particular focus on specific sub-groups in the male population – the young and the socially isolated – men who are perceived as presenting the highest risk to the public.

In summary, then, two sociological perspectives have been proposed to account for recent gender-specific changes in men-tal heath statistics – the increasing visibility of men, particularly young men. It is with these theoretical explanations in mind that the following case study focuses on both gender and age differ-ences in bed occupancy in mental health facilities in England and Wales, the largest constituent part of the UK.

The aim of the case study is to see if the changing gender patterns in the use of mental health services that have emerged in the USA are also evident in the UK. In other words, are men becoming more visible in statistics on mental health service use and is this particularly the case among young men? The data presented in Chapter 7 provide some support for this proposi-tion. Based on an investigation of regional differences in the gender balance of the population in mental health facilities (hospitals and residential care units), the results suggest that, at least as far as England and Wales are concerned, it is men, and not women, who now predominate in these facilities. To what extent, however, is this particularly the case among young men? In other words, as the proportion of men has increased in mental health facilities, have young men become more at risk of institu-tionalisation than have older men?

In a similar way to previous investigations, the case study is based on a detailed exploration of census data on the population in residential mental health facilities in England and Wales for seven census periods in the twentieth century – 1921, 1931, 1951, 1961, 1971, 1981, 1991. These facilities include all psychiatric hospitals and psychiatric units in general hospitals (NHS and the independent sector), and all residential homes and hostels (all sectors – public, commercial and non-profit) officially designated as mental health units. Although bed numbers have been reduced in hospitals, they still form the bulk of this provision a situation quite different from that in relation to physical health care. The specific questions addressed in this case study are as follows:

(1) Are men, rather than women, beginning to dominate in the population using institution-based mental health care in England and Wales?

(2) Within the male sub-population using these services, are younger men more visible than older men?

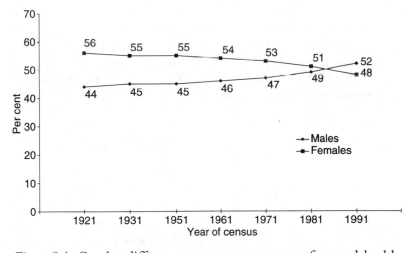

Figure 8.1 Gender differences among occupants of mental health beds in England and Wales, 1921–91

Source: England & Wales Census, 1921, 1931, 1951, 1961, 1971, 1981 and 1991.

Gender trends reversed – men replacing women

Figure 8.1 confirms our previous analysis in Chapter 7, that there is clear evidence of a changing gender trend in the use of residential mental health facilities. In keeping with the traditional stereotype, women outnumbered men in mental health facilities for most of the twentieth century, but in the last decade, this seemingly stable pattern of female dominance was reversed. In 1991, for the first time in the twentieth century, there were more men within these facilities than there were women. In that year, males formed 52 per cent of this population, with females forming 48 per cent – a gender gap of four per cent. Thus, using bed occupancy as a measure of psychiatric diagnosis and treatment, it is clear that men in England and Wales have become increasingly vulnerable to the diagnosis of mental disorder.

What is even more interesting, however, is the fact that this reversal in the gender pattern was not a sudden change in trend. As the data in Figure 8.1 clearly show, the decrease in the proportion of women, and the corresponding increase in the proportion of men, was a steady trend throughout the century. Between 1921 and 1991, as the proportion of women decreased steadily – from 56 per cent to 48 per cent, the proportion of men increased from 44 per cent to 52 per cent – an increase of eight percentage points. This means that as the twentieth century ended and the twenty-first began, 'madness' emerged as a male rather than a female characteristic. This is not an entirely new phenomenon historically, as the image of 'madness' in the seventeenth and eighteenth centuries was male. The artists of the time presented the world with pictures of the 'lunatic' as a man in chains – physically restrained for the safety of himself and others (for historical discussion, see Porter, 1987).

This trend towards an increase in the number of men using institution-based mental health services is also confirmed when the information on bed occupancy is estimated in a different way – in terms of the general population, rather than in terms of the population in residential mental health facilities. In other words, as shown previously in Chapter 3, the same numbers are again used to calculate how many men and women are in psychi-

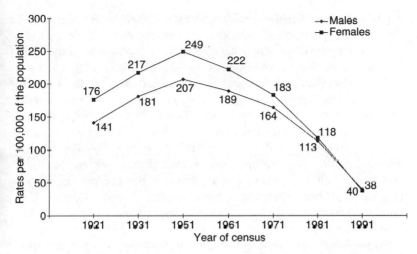

Figure 8.2 Males and females in mental health beds in England and Wales, rates per 100,000 of the population, 1921–91
Source: England & Wales Census: 1921, 1931, 1951, 1961, 1971, 1981 and 1991.

atric facilities as compared to their total numbers – in this case rates per 100,000 – within their respective male and female sub-populations. Figure 8.2 gives this information. The use of population rates gives a more accurate picture of the situation in the context of the wider society, although it has limitations. For example, as with other areas of health, rates of service use are only one indicator of levels of health and illness in society. However, as statistics on mental health service use – especially those relating to hospital treatment – have been widely used in the past to make the case for a high level of 'madness' in the female population, this particular line of argument is worth pursuing here.

When differences in male:female rates of bed occupancy in mental health facilities per 100,000 of the general population are calculated, the growing visibility of men in these facilities is clear (see Figure 8.2). Despite a dramatic overall reduction in the size of the population in mental health facilities – from 120,060 in 1921 to 38,963 in 1991 – males now show higher rates of bed occupancy than females (Prior and Hayes, 2001b). As Figure 8.2 clearly indicates, not only did the gender difference in occupancy rates per 100,000 of the total population decline steadily over the course of the twentieth century – from 35 beds in 1921 to 2 beds in 1991 – but the greatest reduction in the rate of service use occurred among women. For example, while female occupancy rates dropped from an all-time high of 249 beds per 100,000 of the total population in 1951 to just 38 per 100,000 beds in 1991 – a reduction of 211 beds per 100,000 – the equivalent decrease among males was much lower, at only 167 per 100,000. It is this specific trend – the greater decline in the rate of bed occupancy by women – that explains the current predominance of men in residential mental health facilities.

In summary, then, the results of this investigation suggest that there has been a substantial gender reversal in the use of mental health care facilities in England and Wales in the latter part of the twentieth century. Although women featured more prominently than men for much of the century, in 1991, men overtook women in terms of their use of these services. In other words, at least as far as England and Wales are concerned, it may no longer be said that women are higher users of mental health services than are men. In fact, the opposite is now the case in that it is men – and not women – who currently predominate in residential mental health facilities. This finding – or the increasing predominance of men within these facilities – is both consistent with and further confirms recent national and international research in this area (Payne, 1995, 1996; Gijsbers van Wijk *et al.*, 1995; Kessler *et al.*, 1994; Lelliot *et al.*, 1994; Regier *et al.*, 1993).

To what extent, however, can this increasing predominance of men be explained by the disproportionate presence of younger men within these facilities? In other words, as more recent American research on institution-based treatment programmes suggests (see Sanguineti *et al.*, 1996; Reicher-Rossler and Rossler, 1993), is the growth in the male population in these mental health facilities simply a reflection of a disproportionate increase in the numbers of young men? It is with this specific question in mind that the following section focuses on both gender and age.

Table 8.1 Gender differences across the age distribution of bed occupants aged 15 years and over in mental health facilities in England and Wales, 1991

Age	Men (%)	Women (%)	Gender gap (%)	Total (%)
15–24	57	43	14	5.1
25–34	69	31	38	10.3
35–44	68	32	36	10.7
45–54	64	36	28	11.6
55–64	61	39	22	14.7
65+	38	62	−24	47.6
N	19,952	18,686	—	38,638

Source: England & Wales Census, 1991.

Gender and age – the emergence of two distinct populations

The data in Table 8.1 show gender differences in the age distribution of the population in residential mental health facilities in 1991. The following six mutually exclusive age-bands – 15–24 years, 25–34 years, 35–44 years, 45–54 years, 55–64 years, and 65 years or older – are distinguished. If, as the American literature suggests, the explanation for an increasing proportion of men in mental health facilities is related to the specific presence of young men, then we would expect to notice a particular concentration of young men – one not mirrored among young women – in this population.

An overall inspection of the data provides some limited support for this age-specific proposition (see Table 8.1). As the calculation for male-female percentage differences across all age categories clearly shows, in all but one instance – people aged 65 years or older – the proportion of men was consistently higher than that of women. For example, males represented over two-thirds of the

Table 8.2 The gender gap among bed occupants aged 15 years and over in mental health facilities in England and Wales, 1921–81

Age	(Percentage difference: Men − Women)				
	1921	1951	1961	1971	1981
15–24	0	14	18	18	14
25–34	−4	10	16	16	20
35–44	−6	2	12	16	18
45–54	−16	−10	2	12	16
55–64	−18	−20	−12	0	10
65+	−26	−34	−40	−38	−34

Note: Figures could not be included for the 1931 census because of the absence of distinguishing data on age.

Source: England & Wales Census, 1921, 1951, 1961, 1971 and 1981.

population in residential mental health facilities in both the 25–34 and 35–44 year-old age groups in 1991. Similarly, in the 55–64 year-old age group, the male proportion was just slightly lower, at just over three-fifths, or exactly 61 per cent, of the population. This is not to deny, however, that among people aged 65 years or more, women clearly outnumbered men by a significant margin – 62 per cent for women and 38 per cent for men – a gender gap of 24 per cent. It is clear, therefore, that, while there are more men than women in all age categories up to the age of 65 years, the numbers in the two youngest age groups (men aged 15–34 years) are not sufficiently large to argue for a particular vulnerability among younger men. From an overall perspective, this suggests that the higher visibility of younger men in the NLS population (Lelliot et al., 1994) or in admission rates (Payne, 1995, 1996) is not of a sufficient magnitude to make an impact on the overall population in mental health beds.

It is interesting to note that the gender gap across age groups is not new, but dates from the middle of the twentieth century (see Table 8.2). This gender gap, with men predominating, emerged for those aged 15–44 years as early as 1951, among those aged 45–54 years in 1961 and, by 1981, it applied to all

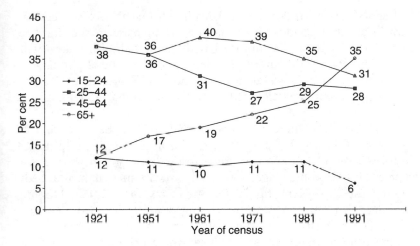

Figure 8.3 Age differences among men aged 15 years and over in mental health beds in England and Wales, 1921–91
Source: England & Wales Census: 1921, 1951, 1961, 1971, 1981 and 1991.

age groups except those over 65 years. What is even more interesting is that this trend – towards the increasing predominance of men among the under-65-year-olds – directly parallels the reduction in psychiatric hospital beds that began in England and Wales in the early 1960s (Jones 1993: 187). It also directly parallels the reduction in the total number of mental health beds in England and Wales – from 120,060 in 1921 to 38,638 in 1991. In other words, as the number of beds available in these facilities decreased, the proportion of men using them increased.

It is clear from our analysis that the increasing mental health care needs of older men cannot be ignored. A further exploration of the data, focusing on age differences within the male subpopulation, showed that men over the age of 65 are currently the group of men most vulnerable to institutionalisation in England and Wales (see Figure 8.3). This group almost trebled as a proportion of the male population in residential mental health facilities between the beginning and the end of the twentieth century – from 12 per cent in 1921 to 35 per cent in 1991. This is in contrast to the percentage of men in the youngest age category (15–24 years), which halved – from 12 to 6 per cent – over the same period. This trend, or the increase in the number of older men in institution-based mental health care, will undoubtedly become more pronounced as the general population continues to age. This situation will, no doubt, present new challenges both for mental health services in general and for those specifically aimed at older people.

However, the increase in older men has to be seen in the context of the whole 'cared-for' population in mental health facilities, where older women continue to predominate. In 1991, there were 11,403 women aged over 65 years in mental health beds while the equivalent figure for men was only 6,989. Despite the fact that older men are increasing numerically in these facilities, the majority of residents will continue to be women for some time to come. In other words, there are now two distinct sub-populations in terms of age and gender in residential mental health facilities in England and Wales – men of working age and women of retirement age. However, this pattern is not so obvious because of the dominance of women among those aged 65 years and over, the age group which now forms almost half (48 per cent) of the total population in institution-based mental health care. This finding adds strength to existing arguments for a greater resourcing of community-based mental health services for older people (Wilson, 2000). As this section of the population increases, due to better physical health and longer life-spans, the full range of mental health care and treatment will need to be made available to them. Otherwise the proportion of older women – and increasingly older men – using costly residential mental health care will continue to rise.

Adjudicating between the two theoretical explanations

As discussed earlier, previous theoretical research suggests two competing explanations – the social causation model versus the social construction model – to account for changing gender patterns in the use of mental health services or, in this case, the increasing visibility of men in institution-based mental health care. The social causation model accounts for this change in terms of an increase in the experience of mental health problems by men, while the social construction model attributes it to a re-conceptualisation of mental disorder which highlights male rather than female problems. The results of this case study, however, provide only limited support for either explanation.

First, in direct confirmation of the expectations of social construction theorists, the proportion of men in mental health facilities has grown substantially over the twentieth century, from 44 per cent in 1921 to a majority position of 52 per cent in 1991. However, this male increase in the cared-for population in mental health facilities is not a universal finding, but varies substantially by age. In fact, the fastest and most consistent increase in the male population within these facilities has not occurred among the young, as predicted by social construction theorists, but among the oldest age category of individuals aged 65 years or older. Between 1921 and 1991, men aged 65 years or older almost trebled as a proportion of the male population in residential mental health facilities – from just 12 per cent in 1921 to 35 per cent in 1991. This is in direct contrast to the youngest age category, where the proportion of men aged 15 to 24 years halved over the same period – from 12 per cent to 6 per cent. Thus, it is increasingly older men, and not younger men, who are most likely to receive institution-based mental health treatment in England and Wales.

Second, although it could be argued that the increasing visibility of men in residential mental health facilities lends some support to the social causation explanation, again the evidence in support of this position is extremely limited. For example, while it could be suggested that this increase – particularly among older men, or those aged 65 years or older – simply reflects an increase in mental health problems in this age group, research undertaken elsewhere calls into question this explanation. In fact, there is no empirical evidence to suggest that there has been a significant increase in the experience of illness among either men or women in this older age group. Rather, the existing evidence points to explanations based on demographic changes (including an ageing population and the weakening of family ties) which result in greater numbers of older people requiring long-term care (for discussion, see Wilson, 2000).

A similar case – some limited evidence particularly in support of the social causation explanation – can also be made in relation to the working-age population. The social causation model, for example, is partly confirmed by the case study in that there is some evidence to suggest an increase in mental health problems among young men. However, research from elsewhere calls into question this interpretation, pointing instead to a rise in the reporting of mental health problems by men and a gender-specific change in patterns of psychiatric service use. What seems to be happening is that, while more men are coming forward for help, women are more successful in accessing community-based mental health services (Pfeiffer *et al.*, 1996; Sartorius *et al.*, 1989). Men, in contrast, are increasingly making use of institution-based treatment (Payne, 1996; Miller, 1993; Reicher-Rossler and Rossler, 1993; Thomas *et al.*, 1993). In other words, it is gender differences in type of treatment accessed, and not a rise in the actual experience of mental health problems among men, that explains these gender differences in the occupancy rates of residential mental health facilities within the working-age population.

On balance, therefore, it looks as if the evidence gives more weight to the idea that there has been a change in the conceptualisation of mental disorder – resulting in higher rates of psychiatric diagnosis and of admission to institution-based mental health care for men. However, the possibility that men are experiencing more mental health problems than previously and that they are now more willing to report these problems should not be dismissed. In the next chapter, these issues will be explored more fully in another area of the UK – Northern Ireland.

What is without doubt, however, is that it is men – and not women – who are currently more likely to receive institution-based mental health care in England and Wales. Although it is true that women outnumbered men in mental health beds for most of the twentieth century, men now occupy a majority position. Furthermore, although the shift from female to male dominance in mental health facilities became visible in statistics only in 1991, it had already begun in the 1950s among the young, and had extended to all age groups under 65 years by 1971. However, because of the dominance of women among those aged 65 years and over, there are currently two distinct sub-populations in residential mental health facilities in England and Wales – men of working-age and women of retirement age.

Summary

- Women were higher users of institution-based mental health care in England and Wales for most of the twentieth century
- The gender trend was reversed in 1991, when, for the first time, men were in the majority in the population in mental health beds in England and Wales
- The reversal of the gender trend is clear for all age groups under the age of 65 years
- There are two distinct sub-populations with different care needs in mental health facilities in England and Wales – working-age men and retired women
- Although women continue to dominate among older people (65 years and over), men form a substantial and increasing proportion of this cared-for population

9 Young Men as Reluctant Help-Seekers

Chapter outline

- Introduction
- Theoretical approaches to explaining mental health statistics in Northern Ireland
- Gender differences in the use of institution-based care
- The emergence of two distinct sub-populations in mental health facilities
- Evaluating the theoretical models
- Summary

Introduction

In the past, young men have not featured prominently in mental health statistics, a fact that contrasts sharply with their high visibility in crime statistics (Daly, 1994). This pattern confirms the accepted view of young men as individuals who show their emotional or psychological problems in acts of violence and other socially unacceptable behaviour, rather than in seeking help from health services. In other words, illness behaviour is not as acceptable for young men as it is for young women (see Shorter, 1990). As we have discussed in Chapters 7 and 8, young men are now becoming more visible in psychiatric statistics in the USA, mainly due to the inclusion of substance dependence and personality disorder in the calculation of these statistics in recent years. In

Chapter 8 we found that this pattern has not yet emerged in England and Wales in one very important area of mental health provision, institution-based care, when overall bed occupancy in mental health facilities was investigated. However, there is some evidence of an increase in young men in admission rates (Payne, 1996, 1995) and in the new long-stay population in psychiatric hospitals (Lelliot *et al.*, 1994).

Of special interest here is the fact that a preliminary analysis of similar statistics on bed occupancy in residential mental health facilities in Northern Ireland showed different gender patterns from those in England and Wales (see Chapter 7, Table 7.2). Based on an investigation of regional differences in the gender balance of the population in mental health facilities, the results suggest that, while men are now in the majority in these facilities in England and Wales, it is women – and not men – who are in the majority in Northern Ireland. Furthermore, there is also some historical evidence to suggest that this predominance of women in institution-based mental health care in Northern Ireland may be a relatively new phenomenon, occurring only in the second half of the twentieth century. As explained in Chapter 7, men predominated as patients in the public asylum system throughout Ireland in the nineteenth century, a pattern that continues to the present day in the Republic of Ireland, which has a different health care system from that in Northern Ireland (see Cleary, 1997; Finnane, 1981). The aim of this chapter, therefore, is to examine gender patterns in the population in mental facilities in Northern Ireland more thoroughly, with a specific focus on young men. This analysis will take place against the background of gender debates in mental health literature, but will also take into account the particular socio-political context of the society being studied.

Northern Ireland, with a history of civil unrest, provides the researcher with a unique opportunity for the study of the relationship between gender and mental health. Since the start of the present political conflict – the 'troubles' – in 1969, over 3,000 people have been killed and almost 42,000 injured in politically-motivated violence (Fay *et al.*, 1999: 159–62; Hayes and McAllister, 1999: 457–9). Furthermore, there is some empirical evidence to suggest that the vast majority of deaths have occurred among young men, most notably males under the age of 35 years (Hayes and McAllister, 2001: 905). Second, although the association between violence and mental health has been extensively investigated in Northern Ireland, the contribution of gender has not been studied to date. Mindful of this omission, the case study presented in this chapter will be placed within the context of two distinct research traditions – the international literature on gender and mental health, as discussed in Chapters 7 and 8, and the nationally-specific literature on war and mental health.

Theoretical models

The literature on the impact of war on mental health belongs within the theoretical framework of the social causation perspective, which suggests that changes in psychiatric statistics are a reflection of changes in the experience of mental health problems. Theorists who apply the social causation perspective argue that there is a direct link between exposure to a war situation and mental illness (see, for example, Hyams *et al.*, 1996; Farhood *et al.*, 1993; Aubrey, 1941). According to this view, both the distress and the social disruption caused by war are key factors in explaining increases in mental illness within a society. More importantly, however, because men have traditionally been the main protagonists in war situations, the theory also implies that men are more susceptible to higher levels of mental illness than women. In other words, it is argued that it is the differential experience of war by men and women that explains the gender gap in mental health statistics in Northern Ireland.

The social construction perspective, in contrast, explains gender differences in mental health statistics in terms of variation in the conceptualisation of mental disorder. As discussed earlier, researchers using this perspective argue that mental health statistics reflect nothing more than changing professional and social views on mental disorder (for discussion, see Chapter 8). More importantly, however, they argue that stereotypical notions of male behaviour, such as their perceived potential for violence towards self and society, have now replaced stereotypical notions of female behaviour in discourses surrounding mental disorder. This, in turn, has led to the growing visibility of men in mental health statistics throughout the western world (see Coontz *et al.*, 1994; Litwack *et al.*, 1993; Miller, 1993).

Past empirical research in Northern Ireland provides only limited support for either explanation. Concentrating initially on the social causation approach – the war model – empirical evidence in support of this theory is mixed. Although some early studies showed an association between civil unrest and an increase in mental illness, the majority suggest little or no such increase resulting from civil disturbances (see Curran, 1988, for a review of this literature). For example, during the period with the highest level of civil unrest, from 1969 to 1974, Fraser (1971) found evidence of 'acute emotional reactions' as well as a general increase in mental illness requiring hospital admission among individuals affected by rioting.

Later research, however, by Cairns and Wilson (1984) calls into question this finding. Using the General Health Questionnaire to examine mild psychiatric morbidity in two specific geographic areas with different levels of recorded violence, this study found little evidence to support a direct association between civil disorder and mental illness. More specifically, the results suggested that, although a small number of people were vulnerable to mental distress, the vast majority remained mentally healthy. This finding was in keeping with international literature on the relationship between mental health and war or civil disorder (see Loughrey and Curran, 1987). Finally, from the few international studies which add gender to the equation, some interesting, if extremely minor, gender-specific differences emerge in the relationship between mental health and war. For example, in the Lebanon, there is some limited empirical evidence to suggest that it is women, and not men, who are more susceptible to mental illness in a war situation (see Farhood *et al.*, 1993; Saigh, 1988).

As pointed out earlier, empirical evidence in support of the social construction model is also mixed. Based predominantly on American findings, there is some evidence to suggest that changes in professional and societal views on mental disorder are impacting on mental health statistics (see Chapters 7 and 8). For example, the inclusion of substance dependence and personality disorder in estimates of psychiatric morbidity in the USA led to a higher lifetime prevalence of mental disorder among men than women (Kessler *et al.*, 1994; Robins and Regier, 1991). In addition, there is evidence in the UK and the USA that young men are increasingly vulnerable not only to the experience of mental disorder, but also to hospitalisation (Payne, 1996, 1995; Sanguineti *et al.*, 1996; Coontz *et al.*, 1994; Lelliot *et al.*, 1994). However, it would be misleading to suggest that this is a universal finding. A number of studies have also shown that women continue to predominate in many psychiatric statistics in the UK and the USA (see Dennerstein, 1995; Pilowsky *et al.*, 1991).

In the context of this research literature, we now present a case study examining gender patterns in the use of institution-based mental health care in Northern Ireland during the twentieth century. Based on the war literature, we would expect the political violence in Northern Ireland to have little effect on the use of mental health services, with the possible exception of increasing the visibility of women. Based on the social constructionist arguments in the mental health literature, we would expect the opposite – an increase in the proportion of men, particularly young men, using these services.

As in previous chapters, this case study is based on a detailed exploration of census data on the population in residential mental health facilities in Northern Ireland for six census periods during the twentieth century – 1926, 1937, 1951, 1971, 1981, 1991. Figures for the seventh census – 1961 – could not be included because of the absence of distinguishing data between physical and mental health facilities. Residential mental health facilities include all psychiatric hospitals and psychiatric units in general hospitals (all are publicly funded in Northern Ireland), and all residential homes and hostels officially designated as mental health facilities (all sectors – public, commercial and non-profit). Although bed numbers have been reduced in hospitals in the second half of the twentieth century, they still form the bulk of provision in terms of mental health care.

In a similar vein to the case study presented in Chapter 8, the aim is to see if the changing gender patterns in the use of mental health services that have emerged in the USA are also evident in Northern Ireland. In other words, are men becoming more visible in psychiatric statistics and is this particularly the case among young men? As we saw earlier, the data presented in Chapter 7 provide little support for this proposition in that it is women, and not men, who currently predominate within these facilities (see Table 7.2). It is important to note, however, that the gender gap – or difference in the proportion of men and women – is quite low in this instance at just two per cent (when the decimal points have been rounded up). In addition, there is some empirical evidence to suggest a slight increase in the proportion of men – from 47 per cent to 49 per cent – in these facilities between 1981 and 1991. It is with these specific findings in mind, that the following case study focuses on gender and age differences in the use of institution-based mental health care in Northern Ireland, during the twentieth century.

Gender trends – a game of musical chairs

As suggested by our analysis in Chapter 7, the data in Figure 9.1 provide clear evidence of a changing gender trend in the use of residential mental health facilities in Northern Ireland. Of

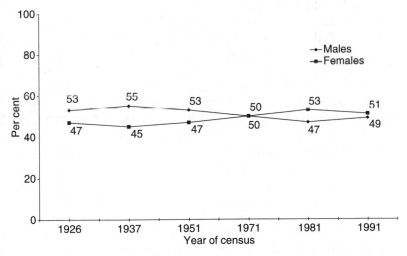

Figure 9.1 Gender differences among bed occupants in mental health facilities in Northern Ireland, 1926–91
Source: Northern Ireland Census, 1926, 1937, 1951, 1971, 1981, 1991.

special interest here is the fact that men were in the majority in institution-based care in Northern Ireland prior to 1971. This contrasted with the traditional stereotype of female predominance in psychiatric statistics confirmed in other areas of the UK. This unusual trend parallels the situation in the Republic of Ireland – which was politically connected to Northern Ireland prior to 1921 – where men have predominated in mental health beds both historically and currently (Cleary, 1997; Finnane, 1981). The largest gender differences, or a gap of 10 percentage points, occurred in Northern Ireland in 1937, when men constituted 55 per cent of the population in residential mental health facilities, as compared to 45 per cent for woman. This pattern of male dominance disappeared in 1971 and was reversed in 1981 when women constituted a majority for the first time. In that year, women occupied 53 per cent of mental health beds, while men occupied 47 per cent, a gender gap of six percentage points. By 1991, although females were still in the majority, the gender trends began to reverse yet again, causing a reduction in the gender gap to just two percentage points, with females occupying only slightly over half – 51 per cent – of all mental health beds in Northern Ireland.

A comparison of male and female rates of bed occupancy per 100,000 of the general population mirrors these findings (see Figure 9.2). For example, prior to 1971, the male rate was higher than the female rate, reaching a peak in 1937 of 223 per 100,000 of the general population for males and 186 per 100,000 for females. Since then, the trend has reversed. In 1981, for example, the rate was 110 for females and 96 for males and, by 1991, the rate for females was 109 as compared to 103 for males. In other words, although the female rate continued to be higher than that for males, the gender gap narrowed due to a slight decrease in the rate among females – from 110 to 109, as compared to a noticeable increase among males – from 96 to 103. Of further interest is the fact that this increase in the male rate – a rise of seven per 100,000 of the general population – occurred in the decade from 1981 to 1991 when the general thrust of mental health policy in Northern Ireland, as elsewhere, was to reduce mental health bed numbers.

It is worth noting, however, that despite this policy thrust, the level of bed occupancy and, therefore, of mental health provision

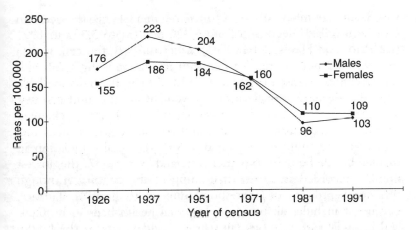

Figure 9.2 Gender differences among occupants of mental health beds in Northern Ireland, rates per 100,000 of the population, 1926–91

Source: Northern Ireland Census, 1926, 1937, 1951, 1971, 1981, 1991.

for both men and women has remained considerably higher in Northern Ireland than in England and Wales. In 1991, the Northern Ireland bed-occupancy rates per 100,000 of the population were well over twice those of their male (103 versus 40) and female (109 versus 38) equivalents in England and Wales (see Chapter 8, Figure 8.2). In other words, men and women with mental health problems in Northern Ireland are more than twice as likely to receive institution-based care than their counterparts in England and Wales. This apparent tendency to over-institutionalise people in Ireland is the subject of a long-running debate that lies outside the scope of the discussion here. In brief, while some researchers argue that it reflects a higher level of mental illness throughout the island of Ireland, others point to a legacy of a high level of institutional provision (in health and welfare) during the nineteenth century (for discussion, Scheper-Hughes, 2001; Walsh and Kendler, 1995).

Despite the comparatively high level of institutionalisation in Northern Ireland, there has also been a dramatic reduction in this type of care in the second half of the twentieth century. In line with developments in mental health care in most of the western world, the number of occupants of mental health beds in Northern Ireland decreased from 5,320 in 1951 to 3,337 in 1991 (see Prior and Hayes, 2001a: 541). Unfortunately, the census data for 1961 did not distinguish between mental and physical health care facilities. Consequently, the 1971 data is the first available after the de-institutionalisation movement of the mid-century. Therefore, it is not clear if the gender trend had already changed before the reduction in bed numbers or at the same time. However, one thing is certain. By 1991, the total population in mental health beds in Northern Ireland was 3,337, the lowest number recorded since the beginning of the century. Although this number does not correspond directly to hospital statistics, because it includes all designated mental health beds in hospitals and in social care facilities (all sectors), evidence from the DHSS (NI) suggests that this is an accurate reflection of the situation at the time. The report on the regional strategy for health and personal social services 1992–7 stated that, at the beginning of the strategy period in 1992, due to an ongoing reduction in the numbers of people in hospital, there were 'approximately 2,000 people in mental health hospitals, who had been there for a year or more' (DHSS (NI), 1992: 45).

In summary, the results of this investigation provide clear evidence of a changing gender trend in the use of residential mental health facilities in Northern Ireland. In contrast to the situation in England and Wales, where women predominated for most of the twentieth century, men were in the majority in institution-based care in Northern Ireland for all census periods prior to 1971. This pattern of male dominance disappeared in 1971 and was reversed in 1981. By 1991, although women were still in the majority, the gender trends began to reverse yet again, causing a reduction in the gender gap to two percentage points, with females occupying only slightly over half, or 51 per cent, of all mental health beds in Northern Ireland. Thus, gender trends in the use of residential mental health facilities in Northern Ireland might well be described light-heartedly as a game of 'musical chairs'.

The question arises, however, as to the extent to which these findings on the gender composition of the population in mental health facilities are similar across all age groups. In other words, are there any important age-specific differences among men and women in their use of institution-based mental health services? For example, are older women more at risk of institutionalisation within the mental health system than either younger women or older men, as is currently the case in England and Wales? Or, alternatively, as suggested by recent research in the USA (see Sanguineti *et al.*, 1996; Reicher-Rossler and Rossler, 1993), are younger men more vulnerable to institution-based treatment than either younger women or older men? With these specific questions in mind, we now investigate gender and age differences in the population in mental health facilities in both 1981 and 1991, the last two census periods of the twentieth century.

Gender and age – the existence of two separate populations

To explore the age-specific differences within the cared-for population, we investigated the age distribution of people within their respective male and female sub-populations in residential mental health facilities for 1981 and 1991. The findings are presented in Figures 9.3 and 9.4. The following six mutually exclusive age-

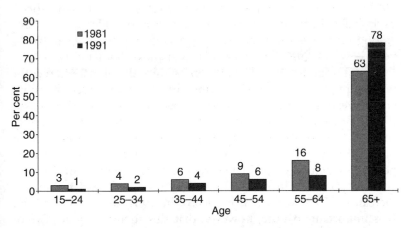

Figure 9.3 Age differences among female occupants of mental health beds in Northern Ireland, 1981–91
Source: Northern Ireland Census, 1981, 1991.

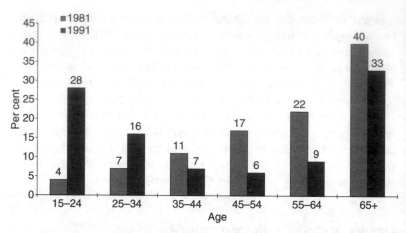

Figure 9.4 Age differences among male occupants of mental health beds in Northern Ireland, 1981–91
Source: Northern Ireland Census, 1981, 1991.

bands are distinguished: 15–24 years, 25–34 years, 35–44 years, 45–54 years, 55–64 years, and 65 years or older. As can be seen clearly from these charts, when the within-population age distributions are compared, men and women show quite different patterns of bed occupancy in residential mental health facilities. Since 1981, increases in bed occupancy among women have been exclusively confined to those aged 65 years or older. In contrast, among men, it is the very young – specifically those aged 15–24 years – whose numbers have increased most dramatically.

Examining the age distribution within the female cared-for population first, the most striking feature is the overwhelming and increasing presence of women over the age of 65 years in this population in both 1981 and 1991 (see Figure 9.3). Women aged 65 years or older constituted 63 per cent of the total female population in residential mental health facilities in 1981, a proportion which rose to 78 per cent – a net increase of 15 percentage points – in 1991. In real terms, this translates into a increase of 277 women, from 1,051 in 1981 to 1,328 in 1991. It is important to note, however, that this increase in the use of secondary care services among older women cannot be understood as simply a by-product of their greater and increasing longevity within the Northern Ireland population as a whole. As revealed in a further analysis of census data, women aged 65 years and older constituted only 19 per cent of the total female adult (aged 15 years or older) population in Northern Ireland in both 1981 and 1991.

This increase in the proportion of women in the older age groups in residential mental health facilities was mirrored by a decrease in the younger age groups. For example, the two youngest groups – women aged 15–34 years – formed a negligible seven per cent of the female sub-population in 1981 and this decreased even further to just three per cent in 1991. In terms of their actual numbers, there were 118 women aged 15–34 years in mental health beds in Northern Ireland on the night of the census in 1981, as compared to just 57 in 1991. A similar pattern of decline is evident in each of the other age groups under 65 years. The proportion decreased from six per cent to four per cent among those aged 35–44 years, and from nine per cent to six per cent for those aged 45–54 years. The most substantial decrease was, surprisingly, in the pre-retirement age group (55–64 years), the proportion of which virtually halved – from sixteen per cent to just eight per cent – in the ten-year period.

Turning now to the male sub-population, the most striking characteristic is its relative youthfulness (see Figure 9.4). The number of men over the age of 35 years decreased as a proportion of the total male sub-population in residential mental health facilities during the 1980s and this pattern was consistent across all of the older age groups. In 1981, for example, men over the age of 65 formed 40 per cent (586 men) of this cared-for population, but, by 1991, it had decreased to 33 per cent (539 men). This reduction in the population of older men in residential mental health care was not reflected in the general population. In fact, the opposite was the case. The general population of men aged 65 years and older actually increased by one per cent – from 13 per cent to 14 per cent – between 1981 and 1991. However, it is clear that this section of the male population – older men – is vastly over-represented in institution-based mental health care.

This is not to deny, however, the substantial increase in the proportion of men, under the age of 35 years, in residential mental health facilities. When taken together, the two youngest

age groups (15–34 years) formed 11 per cent of the male population in these facilities in 1981, but this percentage had risen to
a startling 44 per cent by 1991. In real terms, this translates into
an increase of 547 young men – from 160 in 1981 to 707 in
1991. This growth in the number of young men appears to be a
relatively new phenomenon, becoming apparent only in 1981,
when there was a slight increase in the proportion of men in the
15–34 year age group – from 10 per cent in 1971 to 11 per cent
in 1981. The greatest increase, however, occurred in the proportion of men in the younger of the two age groups (15–24 years),
from just 4 per cent in 1981 to 28 per cent in 1991, or, in
numerical terms, from 64 to 475 men. This proportionate increase
among the young was not mirrored among men aged 35–64
years. In fact, the opposite was the case, with the greatest decrease
occurring among men aged 55–64 years, the pre-retirement age
group.

Thus, it can be concluded that the male population in
institution-based care in Northern Ireland is getting younger and
that the men most vulnerable to admission to this form of care
are those aged 15–34 years. This emerging visibility of young men
in psychiatric statistics is further confirmed in a recent study of
young people, aged 14 to 24 years, who were admitted to adult
psychiatric beds in the acute sector in Northern Ireland between
April 1989 and March 1995. This study not only revealed that
a total of 2,823 young people (aged under 25 years) were
admitted during this period, but that among individuals aged 18
to 24 years (84 per cent of the total) the majority – 57 per cent
– was male (McGilloway *et al.*, 1998: 4).

However, this increase in younger men has to be seen in the
context of the whole 'cared-for' population, where older women
continue to predominate. In 1991, there were 1,328 women aged
over 65 years in residential mental health facilities, while the
equivalent figure for young men, or those aged 15–34 years, was
only 707. In other words, whereas older women constituted 40
per cent of the total cared-for population, the equivalent percentage among young men was slightly under half of that, or just
21 per cent. Despite the fact, therefore, that the number of
younger men in these facilities is increasing, the majority of the
cared-for population will continue to be older women for some
time to come. In other words, similar to England and Wales, there

are now two distinct sub-populations, in terms of age and gender, in residential mental health facilities in Northern Ireland – younger men and older women. However, this pattern is not so obvious because of the dominance of women among those aged 65 years and over, the age group that now forms over half, or 56 per cent, of the total population of both men and women in institution-based mental health care.

Reviewing the explanatory models

As we have already seen, theoretical research suggests two competing explanations – social causation versus social construction – for differences in gender patterns in mental health statistics in Northern Ireland. As explained earlier, whereas social causation theory links political violence to an increase in mental health problems in the population, social construction theory stresses the relationship between changing views on mental disorder and changes in patterns of diagnosis and treatment of mental health problems. The results of this case study suggest that it is the latter, rather than the former, that provides the best theoretical explanation for our findings. The evidence in support of this proposition is threefold.

First, in direct confirmation of the expectations of social construction theorists, young men now form a much greater proportion of the male sub-population in mental health beds in Northern Ireland than ever before. Between 1981 and 1991, the proportion of men, under the age of 35, in institution-based care increased by 33 per cent – from just 11 per cent in 1981 to 44 per cent in 1991. Within this age group, the greatest increase occurred in the proportion of men aged 15–24 years, from just 4 per cent (64 men) in 1981 to 28 per cent (475 men) in 1991. This is in direct contrast to the pattern for young women, where the proportion of those aged 15–24 years within the female cared-for population actually decreased from three per cent in 1981 to a minuscule one per cent in 1991.

Second, this disproportionate increase among young men is occurring at precisely the time when psychiatrists describe the much-reduced acute provision within the mental health care system as so pressurised that it is unsustainable (Kelly, 1998). More importantly, however, indirect evidence from alternative sources suggests that this reduction in bed numbers has been accompanied by a shift in public and professional opinion on mental disorder. To be specific, stereotypical notions of male behaviour, such as their perceived potential for violence towards self and society, are becoming very influential in discourses surrounding mental disorder. As in other areas of the western world, people in Northern Ireland who are perceived as presenting the most risk to society are most likely to be offered institution-based mental health care. The most recent study that examined gender differences in diagnoses among psychiatric patients in Northern Ireland supports this finding. This study found that '[s]ubstance abuse, personality disorder and schizophrenia were more prevalent among young men, while proportionately more of those with neurotic and eating disorders were female' (McGilloway et al., 1998: iii). In other words, the diagnoses attributed to young men are clearly those that are more often associated with dangerous behaviour in the mind of the public, than those attributed to young women.

Finally, it could be suggested that the proportionate increase in the use of mental health beds by women in 1971 – one of the most violent years in Northern Ireland during the twentieth century – lends some empirical support to the social causation approach, which postulates a link between war and mental illness. However, a further examination of the findings suggests otherwise. First, when actual bed numbers are calculated, there was no net increase in the number of women in mental health facilities during this period. Second, as the main actors in civil unrest, the greatest and most immediate impact should have been on the young. However, when the age distribution among females in 1971 was examined, this was not the case. For example, women aged 65 years and over formed the largest proportion (53 per cent) of mental health bed occupants, while women aged 15–34 years were in the minority (6 per cent). Finally, although there is some empirical evidence to suggest that young men may be at increasing risk of mental illness, the changing age pattern in the use of institution-based care did not occur until 1991, nearly twenty-five years after the conflict began. In addition, when these age-specific differences finally did occur, it was young men, and not middle-aged men (who reached adulthood at the onset of the troubles), who emerged as the most vulnerable group.

This is not to suggest, however, that we should dismiss the possibility of long-term damage to the mental health of young people whose lives have been dominated by political strife and civil unrest for the past thirty years. A sevenfold increase in the proportion of young men aged 15–24 years in mental health beds between 1981 and 1991 must raise the issue of the context of these lives. These are the 'sons of the troubles', who were born at the time of the most intensive political violence in Northern Ireland (from 1969 to 1972) and have lived their lives in a society that is highly ambivalent about peace (Hayes and McAllister, 2001). And, although there have been studies on the impact of the political conflict on the lives of the general population in Northern Ireland (see Fay *et al.*, 1999), its specific impact on young people continues to be a neglected area of research. Further and more intensive studies on the actual circumstances of the lives of the 15–24 year old cohort and their younger siblings is clearly needed. This may yield information on the contribution of political conflict to their visibility in the mental health system.

Clearly, it can no longer be argued that young men are absent from psychiatric statistics. The evidence presented here shows that in Northern Ireland, at least, young men are increasingly finding their way into the mental health care system. In other words, it has become more acceptable for them to articulate their emotional and psychological problems in 'illness' terms. Although it cannot be argued that they are now eager to seek help, it seems that they are less reluctant help-seekers than their older brothers. This is not to deny, however, the current predominance of women in mental health facilities. Although men outnumbered women in mental health beds for most of the twentieth century, since 1981, women occupy a slight majority position. Furthermore, because of the dominance of women among those aged 65 years and over, there are currently two distinct sub-populations in residential mental health facilities in Northern Ireland – men of working age and women of retirement age. This is not to deny, however, the increasing vulnerability of men – particularly young men – to institution-based treatment in this society. As the case study clearly shows, since 1981, not only have bed-occupancy rates for men risen much faster than those for women but, within the male sub-population, it is men aged 15–24 years who are currently at most risk of institutionalisation in the mental health care system in Northern Ireland.

Summary

- Although men formed the majority of the population in institution-based mental health care in Northern Ireland for the first half of the twentieth century, since 1981, women occupy a slight majority position
- As is also the case in England and Wales, there are currently two distinct sub-populations in institution-based care in Northern Ireland – men of working age and women of retirement age
- Since 1981, the greatest increase in the male sub-population has occurred among young men, or those aged 15–34 years

Part IV
The Twenty-First Century in Focus

10 The Future

Introduction

One of the main messages coming through from the data presented in previous chapters is that gender is an essential factor that needs to be considered when planning and delivering a health care system. Not only do men and women appear to have different health needs, but they also show quite different patterns of health service usage. However, the question remains: To what extent do these gender-specific patterns of health service use confirm stereotypical assumptions about the differing health care needs of men and women in the UK today? It is with this specific question in mind that this final chapter briefly re-visits gender-specific stereotypical notions of the physical and mental health care needs of the population, in the light of empirical evidence presented earlier in our discussions. Based on this re-evaluation of old and new evidence, we then proceed to discuss our findings more comprehensively in terms of the future health care needs of the total population in the UK. A key factor, which will be considered in this discussion, is the future financial impact of the growing demand for health and social care services, arising from an expanding population of older women.

Evaluating the stereotype – physical health

The academic debate on gender and physical health, which began in Western Europe in the 1970s, has continued since then on both sides of the Atlantic. For most of the time, it has been generally accepted that two seemingly contradictory trends operate simultaneously. These trends are that women demonstrate higher rates of morbidity than men, but men have higher rates of mortality than women. As first mentioned in Chapter 1, they can be summarised in the catchy, if stereotypically based phrase, 'women are sicker but men die quicker'. Here, we review the empirical evidence for this statement, evidence that has already been presented in earlier chapters.

Focusing initially on the first part of the old adage – 'women are sicker' – it is clear that the results of our investigations offer support for this statement. Throughout the UK, women admit to much higher levels of physical illness and make greater use of both primary and secondary health care services than men (see Chapter 4). For example, not only are women significantly more likely than men to report higher levels of illness and have greater contact with their GP, but this gender-differential is maintained when the use of secondary care services is investigated. Throughout the UK, women are much higher users of institution-based treatment (in hospitals and social care units) than are men. In addition, although men predominated during the first part of the twentieth century, women now form the vast majority of the population in residential health and social care facilities, outnumbering men by a ratio of almost three to one. Furthermore, this gender reversal in the use of secondary care services for physical illness and disability has led to the increasing replacement not only of men by women, but of working age men and women by women of retirement age. This is due to the continual expansion of the older female population in all institution-based care. As the results from our two case studies clearly show, it is this factor – the growing and disproportionate concentration of older women, particularly among those aged 85 years or over – which accounts for the ever-increasing predominance of women in the population using secondary care services (see Chapters 5 and 6).

Box 10.1 Women are sicker but most men die quicker

- Women are higher users of both primary and secondary health services than men
- Women now dominate the population in residential health and social care facilities throughout the UK and this is particularly the case among older women
- Although life expectancy rates remain higher among women than among men, when type of illness and age are included in the equation, female mortality rates are now either equivalent to or approximating those of men

---

Turning now to the second component of the old adage – men die quicker – the results of this investigation, however, provide only limited support for the universality of this statement. Although women continue to experience much lower mortality rates than men across a variety of illnesses, the statement that 'men die quicker' is not as clear-cut as originally perceived. First, as explained earlier, while mortality rates are much higher among men than women in relation to certain illness, such as lung or heart disease, this is not a universal finding (see Chapter 4). For example, recent mortality estimates based on diseases of the circulatory system suggest that women are just as likely to die from these diseases as are men. Even among long-standing differential mortality rates, such as deaths arising from heart or lung disease, there is growing evidence to suggest that the gender gap is narrowing over time. Furthermore, when the gender gap in smoking patterns among the young is taken into account, current predictions suggest that, in the near future, women will experience much higher mortality rates from smoking-related diseases than men.

In summary, then, at least as far as physical health is concerned, there is a great deal of empirical evidence to suggest that the old adage, 'women are sicker but men die quicker', no longer applies. In other words, while the first part of the adage is still correct, the second is open to question. We suggest that a more accurate reflection of the current situation in relation to changing gender patterns in physical health in the UK may be encapsulated in the more complex statement, 'women are sicker but most men die quicker'.

Evaluating the stereotype – mental health

Gender differences in the experience of mental disorder and in the use of mental health services have also been the subject of intensive academic research and debate throughout the western world. Until recently, it was widely accepted that women predominated in all statistics on the reporting of mental illness and on the use of services. From this it was inferred that women had more mental health problems than had men. As already discussed, these facts were summarised in the stereotypical notion of women as the 'madder sex'. The evidence presented in earlier chapters, however, cast serious doubt on this notion.

Although women have traditionally admitted to higher levels of mental illness and have made greater use of both primary and secondary mental health care services than have men, there is increasing evidence that this is no longer the case. For example, not only are men becoming increasingly visible in statistics on psychiatric morbidity, but this is particularly the case when previously excluded conditions, such as personality disorder and substance dependency, are part of the analysis (see Chapter 7). More importantly, however, these increasing levels of reported illness among men are now beginning to translate into their greater use of secondary care services within the mental care sector in the UK. As the results of the analysis of census data in Chapter 7 demonstrate, there is now clear evidence of a changing gender trend in the use of residential mental health facilities in the UK. In keeping with the traditional stereotype, women outnumbered men in mental health facilities for most of the twentieth century. However, in the last decade, this seemingly stable pattern of female dominance disappeared. For the first time in the century, men and women became equal users of these services. It can no longer be said, therefore, that women in the UK are higher users of mental health services than are men. Since 1991, men and women have become equal users of this very large section of mental health service provision – institution-based care.

This is not to deny, however, some important regional differences in the gender balance in the population in mental health facilities in the UK. As the results from our case study of England and Wales clearly demonstrate, in 1991, for the first time in the twentieth century, there were more men than women – 52 per cent as compared to 48 per cent – in these facilities (see Chapter 8). It is important to note, however, that the predominance of men is not a universal finding, but varies by age. For example, while men are currently in a majority across all age groups under the age of 65 years, women clearly predominate among the retired population. In the older cared-for population, women outnumber men by a significant margin – a gender gap of 24 per cent in this instance. This is not to deny, however, the growth in the population of older men in institution-based mental health care throughout the century; those aged over 65 years trebled within the male sub-population between 1921 and 1991. Thus, using bed occupancy as a measure of psychiatric diagnosis and treatment, it can be stated categorically that men – particularly older men – have become increasingly vulnerable to mental disorder in England and Wales.

This is not the case, however, in either Scotland or Northern Ireland, where women continue to predominate in institution-based care. In Northern Ireland, however, there is some empirical evidence to suggest that the gender balance in the population of residential mental health facilities is highly volatile and remains strongly mediated by age (see Chapter 9). Although men were in the majority for most of the twentieth century, this pattern of male dominance disappeared in 1971 and was reversed in 1981, when women constituted a majority for the first time. By 1991, although women were still in the majority, the gender trends began to reverse yet again, with women occupying only slightly over half, or 51 per cent, of all mental health beds in Northern Ireland. Furthermore, since 1981, while increases in bed occupancy among women have been exclusively confined to those 65 years or older, among men, it is the very young, specifically those aged 15–24 years, who have increased the most dramatically in numerical and percentage terms. There are now two distinct sub-populations, in terms of age and gender, in residential mental health facilities in Northern Ireland – younger men and older women.

Box 10.2 Madness is no longer a female malady

- Men are becoming increasingly visible in statistics on psychiatric morbidity and this is particularly the case when previously excluded conditions, such as substance dependence and personality disorder, are included in the analysis
- Men and women are now equal users of secondary mental health care services in the UK
- Irrespective of region, women over the age of 65 years dominate in the female population in institution-based mental health care in the UK
- While men of working age predominate within the male population in institution-based care in England and Wales, it is young men – particularly those aged 15–24 years – who are increasingly finding their way into this type of care in Northern Ireland

---

In summary, then, there is sufficient empirical evidence to reject the stereotypical view of women as the 'madder sex'. Rather, a more accurate reflection of current changing gender patterns in mental health care in the UK might be characterised by the phrase inspired by the pioneering work of the feminist historian, Elaine Showalter (1987) – 'madness is no longer a female malady'.

It is with these changing gender patterns in both physical and mental health in mind, that the following discussions focus on the financial implications of the future health care needs of the total population (male and female) of the UK at the beginning of the twenty-first century.

Financing health care systems – the UK in comparative perspective

One of the most fundamental questions facing any government is how best to resource a health care system that will meet the needs of the entire population and will not place an undue burden on either individuals who are ill or the taxpayer. Governments adopt different solutions when faced with this question – ranging from one that is totally reliant on public funding to one that is totally reliant on private funding, with varying models of financing between these two extremes.

Since 1948, the UK has opted for a model of publicly-funded health care, providing universal cover that is free to all citizens at the point of access (see Chapter 3). In the expectation that the health of the nation would gradually improve, a key underlying assumption at the time of the introduction of the NHS in 1948, was that a publicly-funded health care system would not put an inordinate burden on the public purse. This expectation was not fulfilled. Health expenditure rose steadily from £437 million in 1949 to £2,220 million (at 1949 prices) in 1996. This translated into a real increase, not only in terms of the actual amount of money spent, but also in terms of the percentage of gross domestic product (GDP) allocated to health, which rose from 3.5 per cent in 1949 to 6 per cent in 1996 (Ham, 1999: 73).

However, when compared with other OECD countries, the UK does not overspend on health – Australia spends almost 9 per cent of GDP, the USA about 14 per cent, and the European Union (EU) average is around 8 per cent (see Ham, 1999: 72–80; Baggott, 1998: 160–87; Appleby, 1992). In other words, the UK has a lower level of health expenditure, when considered in terms

of its GDP, than many other countries in a similar economic position. However, one of the main differences is that in the UK most
of this expenditure is publicly funded. In 1975, only 9 per cent
of total health expenditure in the UK was privately funded,
although it rose steadily in the following two decades, so that, by
1996, it had reached 16 per cent (Baggott, 1998: 165; OECD,
1996).

This is in contrast to many other OECD countries, which
resource a much higher percentage of their health expenditure
from private funds – mostly private health insurance schemes. For
example, over 50 per cent of health expenditure in the USA is
privately funded, over 30 per cent in Austria, Switzerland and
Australia, and between 25 and 30 per cent in France, Germany,
Canada, Japan and the Netherlands (Baggott, 1998: 128). The
involvement of private funding leads to different models of health
care provision in these countries – with some opting for parallel
private and public services, some providing private services within
the public health system and others providing public services
within a private health system. However, regardless of the model
of service provision, the existence of a private health care system
in a country inevitably increases inequalities in health, as shown
most clearly in the two-tier system of health care in the USA
(Baggott, 1998: 172–4).

One of the advantages of the availability of private funds for
health care is the possibility of increasing services without financial damage to other areas of public expenditure. In contrast, in
countries such as the UK, where the major source of funding for
health care is general taxation and the National Insurance scheme,
any expansion or contraction of health expenditure has an impact
on other areas of public expenditure. All of the UK governments
throughout the twentieth century have been conscious of the
implications of rising health costs. The statistics on bed occupancy
presented in earlier chapters, are extremely important in any discussion of costs of health care, as the bulk of health expenditure
is on hospital and residential care services (for discussion, see
Ham, 1999: 77–8; Appleby, 1992). Capital expenditure on build-
ings and equipment and current expenditure on staff salaries are
the two largest items on the budget. These are also the areas of
expenditure that are very difficult to curtail, even when hospitals
are closing or reducing in size. It is with this specific issue in

mind – the financial implications of the growth in demand for residential health and social care services – that the following section focuses on the physical health care sector.

Implications of new trends for a publicly-funded health care system

One of the major trends to emerge from the analysis of census data on bed occupancy in hospitals and social care facilities (for physical illness and disability) is that the level of occupancy has increased steadily. This is in spite of a brief downturn during the 1970s and of the increasing use of day-surgery and day-treatment during the 1980s. In 1991, although the provision of day-treatment and day-care continued to increase, the size of the resident (overnight) population in these facilities rose dramatically to its highest point ever during the twentieth century – to 510,165 people (see Chapter 4). This is in direct contrast to the mental health care sector, where the total population in mental health beds plummeted from a high of 223,250 in 1951 to less than a quarter of this size in 1991 – to 52,379 people (see Chapter 7). The current UK government will have to face this challenge, a growing demand for more beds in the physical health care sector. One solution, already applied in the mental health care sector in the 1970s, could be to place a moratorium on any further expansion in institution-based treatment and initiate a radical shift of focus to community-based services. However, this is very unlikely to happen, as it would require the wholesale closure of publicly-funded hospitals and social care facilities – an act of political suicide for any government. The other solution is to find a new source of funding – either through a health tax or through private health insurance – the former leading to higher health costs for the whole population and the latter to higher costs for individuals requiring care.

However, to use the word 'individual' is to neutralise a situation that is anything but neutral. As we have seen in Chapter 6, the increase in the population using hospitals and care facilities has been highly gendered. The bulk (72 per cent) of the 510,165 occupants of health and social care beds designated for physical illness and disability in the UK in 1991 were women, among whom 88 per cent were over the age of 65 years. In theory, men and women are expected to make an equal contribution to the cost of their care, but this is unlikely to occur now, or in the near future, for the following reason. Most systems of health insurance, whether public or private, are administered through employers and therefore are dependent on participation in the workforce. Furthermore, any future health tax is likely to be related either to wealth or to earnings. However, because women have had both an unequal share of wealth and lower earning power than men during the twentieth century, the likelihood that they will be able to fund their own care, either through private insurance or public taxation, is extremely low (for discussion, see Cabinet Office, 2000). This is particularly the case among those approaching old age in the next twenty-five years. In other words, to provide adequate funding for the health and social care needs of the population during the first quarter of the twenty-first century, there would need to be a substantial and immediate redistribution of wealth from men to women. In addition, a transfer of funds would be required, not from the public to the private purse as in the past, but from the private sector to public care, a highly unlikely development. However, there is an alternative solution available – an increasing role for the private sector in health care provision – the feasibility of which is discussed below.

An alternative solution – the private sector

As discussed in Chapters 2 and 3, the idea of a comprehensive and publicly-funded health care system was introduced in 1948 against a background of a public perception that the previous system was not working. This system was a mixture of services – mainly institution-based – run by a diverse group of providers, comprising public, commercial and charitable bodies. The Conservative governments of the 1980s and 1990s, with Margaret Thatcher and John Major as Prime Ministers, re-introduced the idea of having a mixture of private as well as public provision for health and social care services under the new umbrella term of 'a mixed economy of care'. In other words, the commitment to having the public sector as the sole or majority provider of health and social care services lasted for only thirty years.

Since the late 1970s, the incentives offered to the newly-named 'independent sector' (profit and non-profit organisations and companies) have increased the scope of this sector within the total picture of health care in the UK. Some of the incentives were later removed as they were found to be too costly, due to the fact that commercial providers within the independent sector made use of public funding to expand their own, very profitable, empires. The most costly of these (to the public purse) was the perverse incentive within the social security system in the 1980s, which led to an explosion of nursing homes and residential social care facilities. The increase in public expenditure was due to the ease with which individuals could apply for, and be granted, the full costs of residential nursing or social care. During the period in which the incentive existed, 'social security expenditure on residential care for the elderly rose dramatically from less than £20 million in 1980 to around £700 million by the end of the decade' (Baggott, 1998: 232). As a result of this injection of funds, there was a great expansion in commercially-run nursing homes and social care homes. In contrast, the voluntary sector share of residential care remained virtually static – going from 10 per cent in 1980 to 12 per cent in 1990 – while public sector provision almost halved – from 43 per cent to 23 per cent – over this ten-year period (Baggott, 1998: 232; Laing, 1996).

The incentive within the social security system that led to this expansion in the private sector was removed in the *NHS and Community Care Act 1990* in England and Wales, and in similar legislation one year later in Scotland and Northern Ireland. However, in spite of this, commercial provision continued to expand in this area of care. As we saw in Chapter 6, the demand for care from the people who constituted the highest users of residential care – older women – was becoming increasingly focused on the social care sector rather than on the health care sector. Between 1971 and 1991, the female population within the social care sector almost trebled, from 110,102 to 294,782, with this sector providing approximately 90 per cent of all care for older women. This is in direct contrast to the female population in the health sector (hospitals and nursing homes), which experienced a dramatic decline over the same period – from 92,354 in 1971 to 26,555 in 1991.

This demand for services within the social care sector continued to rise during the 1990s and the public sector, which had already closed, or transferred many of its residential social care facilities to the independent sector (profit and non-profit), was in no position to meet it. In contrast, the commercial sector, with plenty of providers ready to meet this demand, was funded once again from public money for many of the new residents. As Laing (1996) explains, this sector which, in 1989, had provided 46 per cent of total nursing and social care beds, had increased its holdings to 64 per cent of these beds by 1996. However, although the provision was delivered within the commercial (private) sector, 60 per cent of the funding came from the public purse. Therefore, as in other OECD countries, although the private sector may have dominated in this area of service delivery in terms of provision, in the UK, the costs of providing such care is still heavily reliant on public funding. The main beneficiaries of this public investment have been older women. It is to this specific issue – the health care needs of an expanding older and predominantly female population – that we now turn.

The special needs of an ageing population

One of the most important factors in the increasing demand and, consequently, the increasing costs of the health care system in the UK at the beginning of the twenty-first century, is the growing demand from an ageing population. Although acute hospital care, catering mainly for people of working age, is the most expensive due to the high costs of medical technology and medical expertise, it accounts for a relatively small proportion of publicly-funded health expenditure. There are two reasons for this.

First, younger people are lower users of health services – in terms of number of visits and duration of treatment – than older people (Charlton and Murphy, 1997a, 1997b; Bruster *et al.*, 1994). This low level of use among the young was confirmed in the census data on bed occupancy in health and social care facilities in the last three decades of the twentieth century. In fact, the proportion of individuals aged 15–64 years in these facilities nearly halved – from 31 per cent to 18 per cent – between 1971 and 1991 (see Chapter 6). Second, working-age people are now more likely than ever to be covered by private health insurance than are older people, because employers increasingly offer it as a fringe benefit (Ham, 1999: 34; Baggott, 1998: 165). Thus, without under-estimating the cost of care for the working-age population, it may be concluded that this cost may decrease, rather than increase, in terms of demands on the public purse, as more young people buy private health insurance. In contrast, the older population (those aged over 65 years) is likely to continue to make increasing demands on the health care system and is less likely to be able to make a substantial contribution to the costs incurred. As already discussed, this is due to the fact that the greatest demand will come from older women, many of whom will be on low incomes (for further discussion, see Cabinet Office, 2000).

Of course, the impact of an ageing population on the UK health care system is not merely confined to cost – it also influences patterns of service demand. At present, women have an average life span of 80 years and men one of 75 years. However, the average life span is continuing to increase and with it the number of people in the 'older old' age category among both men and women. Although older people (mainly women) form the majority of the population in institution-based care for both physical and mental health, an increasing number of both men and women in their seventies and eighties are successfully living independently for longer. For example, whereas in 1971, only 37 per cent of women over the age of 75 were living in private households, by 1991, this proportion had increased to 46 per cent (see Chapter 6). In other words, although the majority of the older female population that are living independently are aged between 65 and 74 years, since 1971, there has also been a notable increase in the proportion of women over the age of 75 living in private households.

These people need access to high quality medical treatment – including surgical and technological innovations – to enable them to maintain their independence for as long as possible. They require, at the very least, access to hip replacement surgery, heart surgery, cataract treatment, physiotherapy services and domiciliary support services (for discussion, see Wilson, 2000). They also require an increase in the resources devoted to research on causes and preventive measures for such debilitating illnesses as dementia, osteoporosis and other conditions associated with old age. In addition, the system will have to take into account the low-cost and long-term health and social care needs of the 5 or 6 per cent of the over-65-year-old population who will require institution-based care.

Institution-based treatment – care or control?

So far in this book, we have not challenged the assumption that the care provided in residential health and social care facilities in the UK during the twentieth century was helpful to the individuals receiving that care. However, as we know from the literature on institutionalisation (Cohen and Scull, 1983; Goffman, 1961; Barton, 1959), this is not always the case. Institution-based care and treatment has been used by society in the past to isolate and exclude certain sections of the population – older people, people with learning and physical disabilities, and people with mental illnesses. As shown in Chapter 3, the level of institutionalisation, when measured in terms of the population in health and social care facilities, increased fairly steadily from the early twentieth century until 1971, but since then has decreased, due mainly to the new emphasis on care in the community. The aim of community care policies, in ideological terms, was to ensure that nobody should be in an institution (whether a hospital or care facility) if the care or treatment could be delivered elsewhere. This shift in perspective was due to the growing realisation during the twentieth century that institutionalisation might be the easy answer for society, but that it is not always the right answer for the individual concerned. 'Care' can easily become 'control' if people are confined to institutions for too long (Conrad, 1997; Conrad and Schneider, 1980; Jones and Fowles, 1984).

This is most clearly seen in mental health policies and mental health care. For the first half of the twentieth century, it was taken for granted that hospital care was the best care for people with chronic mental health problems, some of which were serious and some not. This was shown in the census statistics on bed occupancy in health and social care facilities discussed in Chapter 3. In other words, as the size of the cared-for population increased between 1921 and 1951 – from 491,208 to 603,854 – so too did the proportion of this population – from 28 per cent to 37 per cent – in mental health facilities. Medical advances (including the availability of new drugs) during the 1950s made treatment outside of institutions possible, while sociological research made treatment within institutions questionable. Consequently, during the 1970s and 1980s, there was general agreement between health professionals, policy-makers, politicians and the public at large, that institution-based treatment for mental health problems should be just a small part of a comprehensive mental health service. As a result of this shift in political and professional perception, accompanied by a commitment to change, the population in mental health facilities in the UK dropped from a high of 223,250 in 1951 to a low of 52,379 in 1991 (see Chapter 7). In other words, the population in these facilities is now less than one-quarter of its size in the middle of the twentieth century.

This is not to say that there are fewer people with mental health problems in society, but rather that the primary mode of treatment is no longer institution-based. However, this radical decrease in the population in mental health facilities and in the number of mental health beds available has not occurred without criticism. In the late 1990s, this criticism was expressed by a growing number of mental health service users who demanded more hospital-based care and treatment, and by a section of the public who feared the danger associated with mental disorder. The fears of the public – sometimes described as a moral panic – were mirrored in the mental health White Paper of the Blair Labour Government – *Modernising Mental Health Services: Safe, Sound and Supportive* (DoH, 1998b). This White Paper and the proposed changes in the mental health law, emphasise the need for a safe society and for the monitoring and containment of individuals who are seen as a risk to the public.

As discussed in Chapters 7 and 8, this can lead to an undue focus on certain sections of the population, who are seen to present a higher public risk than others. These are likely to be men rather than women, the young rather than the old, and members of an ethnic minority. If, as is happening in the USA, the fear of the public translates into a tendency to over-institutionalise young men with mental disorders, this will mean that, once again, one section of the health care system will be used for control rather than care. As shown in the case studies presented in Chapters 8 and 9, this trend has already begun to appear in Northern Ireland, although it is not present in any other region of the UK. As yet it is not clear if this trend is unique to

Northern Ireland because of socio-political factors, or if it will appear elsewhere in the UK in the near future, due to changes in public perceptions of certain forms of mental disorder (Payne, 1996; Lelliot *et al.*, 1994; Miller, 1993). If the latter is the case, then mental health services will need to be more accessible and more suitable for men, particularly young men, than they are at present.

What is clear from our discussions, however, is that new gender patterns in service use are emerging in relation to both physical and mental health across the UK. Men, especially younger men, now seem more vulnerable to mental health problems than are women. However, women are more vulnerable to physical health problems than are men, a pattern that is increasingly reflected in mortality rates. It is to these two factors – the changing mortality rates for women and the changing psychiatric morbidity rates for men – that politicians and health care planners should now direct attention.

Summary

- Plans for a twenty-first century health care system need to be based on information on current trends in service use
- The funding of health and social care provision remains problematic, as the demand for institution-based care continues to increase
- The role of the private sector in funding and providing care, especially in the social care sector, needs to be carefully monitored to prevent misuse of public funds
- An ageing population will require a broad range of health and social care services to enable the majority of older people to live independently in their own homes
- Neglected in the past, the mental health care needs of men – particularly young men – need to be considered by health planners in relation to future health care provision in the UK

Bibliography

Abel-Smith, B. (1994) *An Introduction to Health: Policy, Planning and Financing*, London: Longamn.

Allsop, J. (1984) *Health Policy and the National Health Service*, London: Longman.

Annandale, E. and Hunt, K. (eds) (2000) *Gender Inequalities in Health*, Buckingham: Open University Press.

Appleby, J. (1992) *Financing Health Care in the 1990s*, Buckingham: Open University Press.

Arber, S. (1997) 'Comparing Inequalities in Women's and Men's Health: Britain in the 1990s', *Social Science and Medicine*, 44: 773–87.

Arber, S. and Cooper, H. (1999) 'Gender Differences in Health in Later Life: The New Paradox?', *Social Science and Medicine*, 48: 61–76.

Ashton, H. (1991) 'Psychotropic-drug Prescribing for Women', *British Journal of Psychiatry*, 158 (Suppl. 10): 30–5.

Aubrey, L. (1941) 'Incidence of Neurosis in England Under War Conditions', *Lancet*, 2: 175–83.

Baggott, R. (1998) *Health and Health Care in Britain,* 2nd edn, London: Macmillan.

Balarajan, R. (1991) 'Ethnic Differences: Mortality from Ischaemic Heart Disease and Cerebrovascular Disease in England and Wales', *British Medical Journal*, 302: 560–4.

Bartley, M., Popay, J. and Plewis, I. (1992) 'Domestic Conditions, Paid Employment and Women's Experience of Ill-health', *Sociology of Health and Illness*, 14: 313–43.

Bartley, M., Saker, A., Firth, D. and Fitzpatrick, R. (1999) 'Social Position, Social Roles and Women's Health in England: Changing Relationships 1984–1993', *Social Science and Medicine*, 48: 99–115.

Barton, W.R. (1959) *Institutional Neurosis*, Bristol: John Wright & Sons.

Bebbington, P., Dean, C., Der, G., Hurry, J. and Tennant, C. (1991) 'Gender, Parity and the Prevalence of Minor Affective Disorder', *British Journal of Psychiatry*, 158: 40–5.

Bebbington, P., Dunn, G., Jenkins, R., Lewis, G., Brugha, T., Farrell, M. and Meltzer, H. (1998) 'The Influence of Age and Sex on the Prevalence of Depressive Conditions: Report from the National Survey of Psychiatric Morbidity', *Psychological Medicine*, 28: 9–19.

Bebbington, P., Feeney, S., Flannigan, C., Glover, G., Lewis, S. and Wing, J. (1994) 'Inner London Collaborative Audit of Admissions in Two Health Districts:

II. Ethnicity and the Use of the Mental Health Act', *British Journal of Psychiatry*, 165: 743–9.

Bernard, M. and Phillips, J. (eds) (1998) *The Social Policy of Old Age*, London: Centre for Policy on Ageing.

Blaxter, M. (1990) *Health and Lifestyles*, London: Tavistock/Routledge.

Bruster, S., Jarman, B., Bosanquet, N., Weston, D., Erens, R. and Delbanco, T. (1994) 'National Survey of Hospital Patients', *British Medical Journal*, 309: 1542–9.

Bunting, J. (1997) 'Morbidity and Health Related Behaviour of Adults: A Review', in F. Drever and M. Whitehead (eds) *Health Inequalities*, London: Stationery Office, pp. 198–221.

Busfield, J. (1994) 'Is Mental Illness a Female Malady? Men, Women and Madness in Nineteenth Century England', *Sociology*, 28: 259–77.

Busfield, J. (1996) *Men, Women and Madness: Understanding Gender and Mental Disorder*, London: Macmillan.

Busfield, J. (1999) 'Mental Health Policy: Making Gender and Ethnicity Visible', *Policy and Politics*, 27: 57–73.

Busfield, J. (2000) *Health and Health Care in Modern Britain*, Oxford: Oxford University Press.

Cabinet Office (2000) *Women's Income Over a Lifetime: A Report to the Women's Unit*, London: Stationery Office.

Cairns, E. and Wilson, R. (1984) 'The Impact of Political Violence on Mild Psychiatric Morbidity in Northern Ireland', *British Journal of Psychiatry*, 145: 631–5.

Carstairs, V. and Morris, R. (1991) *Deprivation and Health in Scotland*, Aberdeen: Aberdeen University Press.

Charlton, J. and Murphy, M. (eds) (1997a) *The Health of Adult Britain 1841–1994, Vol. 1*, London: Stationery Office.

Charlton, J. and Murphy, M. (eds) (1997b) *The Health of Adult Britain 1841–1994, Vol. 2*, London: Stationery Office.

Cleary, A. (1997) 'Gender Differences in Mental Health', in A. Cleary and M. Treacy (eds) *The Sociology of Health and Illness in Ireland*, Dublin: University College Dublin Press, pp. 193–207.

Cohen, S. and Scull, A. (eds) (1983) *Social Control and the State: Historical and Comparative Essays*, Oxford: Martin Robertson.

Compton, P. (1993) 'Population Censuses in Northern Ireland: 1926–1991', in A. Dale and C. Marsh (eds), *The 1991 Census User's Guide*, London: HMSO, pp. 330–51.

Connell, R. (1995) *Masculinities*, Oxford: Polity Press.

Conrad, P. (ed.) (1997) *The Sociology of Health and Illness: Critical Perspectives*, 5th edn, New York: St. Martin's Press.

Conrad, P. and Schneider, J. (1980) *Deviance and Medicalization: From Badness to Sickness*, St. Louis: CV Mosby.

Coontz, P., Lidz, C. and Mulvey, E. (1994) 'Gender and the Assessment of Dangerousness in the Psychiatric Emergency Room', *International Journal of Law and Psychiatry*, 17(4): 369–76.

Courtenay, W.H. (2000) 'Constructions of Masculinity and Their Influence on Men's Wellbeing: A Theory of Gender and Health', *Social Science and Medicine*, 50: 1385–401.

Curran, P. (1988) 'Psychiatric Aspects of Terrorist Violence: Northern Ireland 1969–87', *British Journal of Psychiatry*, 153: 470–5.

Dale, A. and Marsh, C. (eds) (1993) *The 1991 Census User's Guide*, London: HMSO.

Daly, K. (1994) *Gender, Crime and Punishment*, New Haven, CT: Yale University Press.

Daly, M. (1984) *Gyn/ecology: The Metaethics of Radical Feminism*, London: Women's Press.

David, D. and Brannon, R. (eds) (1976) *The Forty Nine Percent Majority: The Male Sex Role*, Reading, MA: Addison-Wesley.

Dennerstein, L. (1995) 'Mental Health, Work and Gender', *International Journal of Health Services*, 25(3): 503–9.

DHSS (NI) (1992) *Health and Personal Social Services in Northern Ireland: A Regional Strategy 1992–1997*, Belfast: DHSS.

Digby, A. (1999) *The Evolution of British General Practice*, Oxford: Clarendon Press.

DoH (Department of Health) (1996) *On the State of Public Health 1995: Report of the Chief Medical Officer*, London: HMSO.

DoH (Department of Health) (1998a) *Our Healthier Nation (Labour's Strategy)*, London: HMSO.

DoH (Department of Health) (1998b) *Modernising Mental Health Services: Safe, Sound and Supportive*, White Paper, London: HMSO.

DoH (Department of Health) (2000) *Hospital In-patient data 1999–2000*, London: HMSO. Also available on the DoH website at www.doh.gov.uk.

Dohrenwend, B. (1975) 'Sociocultural and Social Psychological Factors in the Genesis of Mental Disorders', *Journal of Health and Social Behaviour*, 16: 365–92.

Doyal, L. (1979) *The Political Economy of Health*, London: Pluto.

Doyal, L. (1995) *What Makes Women Sick?*, London: Macmillan.

Doyal, L. (ed) (1998) *Women and Health Services: An Agenda for Change*. Buckingham: Open University Press.

Doyal, L. (2000) 'Gender Equity in Health: Debates and Dilemmas', *Social Science and Medicine*, 51: 931–9.

Drever, F. and Whitehead, M. (eds) (1997) *Health Inequalities*, London: Stationery Office.

DSM III (1981) *Diagnostic Statistical Manual, Revised Version 3*, Washington DC: American Association of Psychiatry.

Edley, N. and Wetherell, M. (1995) *Men in Perspective: Practice, Power and Identity*, London: Prentice Hall/Harvester Wheatsheaf.

Emslie, G., Hunt, K., Macintyre, S. (1999) 'Problematizing Gender, Work and Health: The Relationship between Gender, Occupational Grade, Working Conditions and Minor Morbidity in Full-time Bank Employees', *Social Science and Medicine*, 48: 33–48.

Evandrou, M. (ed) (1997) *Baby Boomers: Ageing in the 21st Century*, London: Age Concern, England.

Farhood, L., Zubayk, H., Chaya, M., Saadeh, F., Meshefedhan, G. and Sidani, T. (1993) 'The Impact of War on the Physical and Mental Health of the Family: The Lebanese Experience', *Social Science and Medicine*, 36(12): 1555–67.

Fay, M.T., Morrissey, M. and Smyth, M. (1999) *Northern Ireland Troubles*, London: Pluto Press.

Finnane, M. (1981) *Insanity and the Insane in Post Famine Ireland*, London: Croom Helm.

Flannigan, C., Glover, G., Feeney, S., Wing, J., Bebbington, P. and Lewis, S. (1994a) 'Inner London Collaborative Audit of Admissions in Two Health Districts. I: Introduction, Methods and Preliminary Findings', *British Journal of Psychiatry*, 165: 734–42.

Flannigan, C., Glover, G., Wing, J., Lewis, S., Bebbington, P. and Feeney, S. (1994b) Inner London Collaborative Audit of Admissions in Two Health Districts. III: Reasons for Acute Admission to Psychiatric Wards', *British Journal of Psychiatry*, 165: 750–9.

Foster, P. (1995) *Women and the Health Care Industry: An Unhealthy Relationship*, Buckingham: The Open University.

Fraser, R. (1971) 'The Cost of Commotion: An Analysis of the Psychiatric Sequelae of the 1969 Riots', *British Journal of Psychiatry*, 118: 257–64.

Gijsbers van Wijk, C., Kolk, A., van den Bosch, W. and van den Hoogen, J. (1995) 'Male and Female Health Problems in General Practice: The Differential Impact of Social Position and Social Roles', *Social Science and Medicine*, 40: 597–611.

Goffman, E. (1961) *Asylums*, New York: Doubleday.

Gomez, J. (1993) *Psychological and Psychiatric Problems in Men*, London: Routledge.

Gove, W. (1973) 'Sex, Marital Status, and Mortality', *American Journal of Sociology*, 79: 45–67.

Gove, W. and Tudor, J. (1973) 'Adult Sex Roles and Mental Illness', *American Journal of Sociology*, 78: 813–35.

Green, D.S. (1987) *The New Right: The Counter Revolution in Political, Economic and Social Thought*, Brighton: Wheatsheaf.

Ham, C. (1999) *Health Policy in Britain*, 4th edn, London: Macmillan.

Harding, S. (1995) 'Social Class Differences in Mortality of Men: Recent Evidence from the OPCS Longitudinal Study', *Population Trends*, 80: 31–7.

Hayes, B.C. and McAllister, I. (1999) 'Generations, Prejudice and Politics in Northern Ireland', in A. Heath, R. Breen and C.T. Whelan (eds) *Ireland North and South: Perspectives from the Social Sciences*, Oxford: Oxford University Press, pp. 457–91.

Hayes, B.C. and McAllister, I. (2001) 'Sowing Dragon's Teeth: Public Support for Political Violence and Paramilitarism in Northern Ireland', *Political Studies*, 49: 901–22.

Hensher, M. and Edwards, N. (1999) 'Hospital Provision, Activity, and Productivity in England Since the 1980s', *British Medical Journal*, 319: 911–14.

HMSO (1956) *Report of the Committee of Enquiry into the Cost of the NHS*, Cmd 9663, London: HMSO. (Guillebaud Committee)

House, J., Landis, K. and Umberson, D. (1988) 'Social Relations and Health', *Science*, 241: 540–5.

Hu, Y. and Goldman, N. (1990) 'Mortality Differentials by Marital Status: An International Comparison', *Demography*, 27: 233–50.

Hunt, K. and Annandale, E. (1999) 'Relocating Gender and Morbidity: Examining Men's and Women's Health in Contemporary Western Societies. Introduction to Special Issue on Gender and Health', *Social Science and Medicine*, 48: 1–5.

Hyams, K., Wignall, F. and Roswell, R. (1996) 'War Syndromes and Their Evaluation: From the US Civil War to the Persian Gulf War (Review)', *Annals of Internal Medicine*, 125(5): 398–405.

Jacobson, B., Smith, A. and Whitehead, M. (1991) *The Nation's Health: A Strategy for the 1990s*, 2nd edn, London: King's Fund Centre.

Jenkins, R., Lewis, G., Bebbington, P., Brugha, T., Farrell, M., Gill, B. and Meltzer, H. (1997) 'The National Psychiatric Morbidity Surveys of Great Britain – Initial Findings from the Household Survey', *Psychological Medicine*, 27: 775–89.

Jenkins, R. and Meltzer, H. (1995) 'The National Survey of Psychiatric Morbidity in Great Britain', *Social Psychiatry and Psychiatric Epidemiology*, 30: 1–4.

Jones, H. (1994) *Health and Society in Twentieth Century Britain*, London: Longman.

Jones, K. (1993) *Asylums and After*, London: Athlone Press.

Jones, K. and Fowles, A.J. (1984) *Ideas on Institutions*, London: Routledge & Kegan Paul.

Kaplan, H. and Sadock, B. (1995) *Comprehensive Textbook of Psychiatry Vol. 1 & 2*, 6th edn, Baltimore: Williams & Wilkins.

Kawachi, I., Kennedy, B.P., Gupta, V. and Prothrow-Smith, D. (1999) 'Women's Status and the Health of Women and Men: A View from the States', *Social Science and Medicine*, 48: 21–32.

Kelly, C.B. (1998) 'An Audit of Acute Psychiatric Admission Bed Occupancy in Northern Ireland', *The Ulster Medical Journal*, 67: 44–8.

Kent, D., Fogarty, M. and Yellowless, P. (1995a) 'A Review of Studies of Heavy Users of Psychiatric Services', *Psychiatric Services*, 46(12): 1247–53.

Kent, D., Fogarty, M. and Yellowless, P. (1995b) 'Heavy Utilization of Inpatient and Outpatient Services in a Public Mental Health Service', *Psychiatric Services*, 46(12): 1254–7.

Kessler, R., McGonigle, K., Zhao, S., Nelson, C., Hughes, M., Eshleman, S., Wittchen, H. and Kendler, K. (1994) 'Lifetime and 12 Month Prevalence of DSM-III-R Psychiatric Disorders in the United States. Results from the National Co-Morbidity Survey', *Archives of General Psychiatry*, 51: 8–19.

Kimmell, M. and Messner, M. (eds) (1995) *Men's Lives*, 3rd edn, Boston: Allyn & Bacon.

Klein, R. (1995) *The New Politics of the NHS*, London: Longman.

Kohler Riessman, C. and Gerstel, N. (1985) 'Marital Dissolution and Health: Do Males or Females Have Greater Risk?', *Social Science and Medicine*, 20: 627–35.

La Fond, J. and Durham, M. (1992) *Back to the Asylum: The Future of Mental Health Law and Policy in the United States*, Oxford: Oxford University Press.

Lahelma, E., Martikainen, P., Rahkonen, O. and Silbentoinen, K. (1999) 'Gender Differences in Ill-health in Finland: Patterns, Magnitude and Change', *Social Science and Medicine*, 48: 7–19.

Laing, R.D. (1960) *The Divided Self: An Existential Study in Sanity and Madness*, London: Tavistock.

Laing, W. (1996) *Laing's Review of Private Health Care 1996*, London: Laing & Buisson.

Le Grand, J. and Bartlett, W. (1993) *Quasi-Markets and Social Policy*, London: Macmillan.

Lelliot, P., Wing, J. and Clifford, P. (1994) 'A National Audit of New Long-Stay Psychiatric Patients 1: Method and Description of the Cohort', *British Journal of Psychiatry*, 165: 160–9.

Litwack, T., Kirschner, S. and Wack, R. (1993) 'The Assessment of Dangerousness and Predictions of Violence: Recent Research and Future Prospects', *Psychiatric Quarterly*, 64(3): 245–73.

Loring, M. and Powell, B. (1988) 'Gender, Race and DSM-III: A Study of the Objectivity of Psychiatric Diagnostic Behavior', *Journal of Health and Social Behavior*, 29: 1–22.

Loughrey, G. and Curran, P. (1987) 'The Psychopathology of Civil Disorder', in A.M. Dawson and G.M. Besser (eds) *Recent Advances in Medicine, No. 20*, Edinburgh and London: Churchill Livingstone, pp. 1–17.

Luck, M., Bamford, M. and Williamson, P. (2000) *Men's Health: Perspectives, Diversity and Paradox*, Oxford: Blackwell Science.

Lyons, R.A., Crome, P., Monaghan, S., Killalea, D. and Daley, J.A. (1997) 'Health Status and Disability among Elderly People in Three UK Districts', *Age and Ageing*, 26: 203–9.

MacDonald, M. (1981) *Mystical Bedlam: Madness, Anxiety and Healing in Seventeenth Century England*, Cambridge: Cambridge University Press.

Macintyre, S. (1986) 'Marriage is Good for Your Health: Or Is It?', *Proceedings of the Royal Philosophical Society of Glasgow*.

Macintyre, S., Ford, G. and Hunt, K. (1999) 'Do Women Over-report Morbidity? Men's and Women's Responses to Structured Prompting on a Standard Question on Long Standing Illness', *Social Science and Medicine*, 48: 89–98.

Macintyre, S., Hunt, K. and Sweeting, H. (1996) 'Gender Differences in Health: Are Things Really As Simple As They Seem?', *Social Science and Medicine*, 42(4): 617–24.

Manning, N. and Shaw, I. (1999) 'Mental Health Policy into the 21st Century', *Policy and Politics*, 27: 5–12.

Marsh, C. (1993) 'An Overview', in A. Dale and C. Marsh (eds) *The 1991 Census User's Guide*, London: HMSO, pp. 1–15.

Mason, P. and Wilkinson, G. (1996) 'The Prevalence of Psychiatric Morbidity: OPCS Survey of Psychiatric Morbidity in Great Britain', *British Journal of Psychiatry*, 168: 1–3.

Maynard, A. and Bloor, K. (1996) 'Introducing a Market to the United Kingdom's NHS', *The New England Journal of Medicine*, 334: 604–8.

McDonough, P. and Walters, V. (2001) 'Gender and Health: Reassessing Patterns and Explanations', *Social Science and Medicine*, 52: 547–59.

McGilloway, S., Scott, D., Merriman, B. and Donnelly, M. (1998) *Admission of Young People to Psychiatric Hospital Care: An Analysis of Routine Data*, Belfast: Health and Social Care Research Unit, Queen's University of Belfast.

McQueen, D. (1987) 'A Research Programme in Lifestyle and Health: Methodological and Theoretical Considerations', *Revue d'Epidemiologie et de Sante Publique*, 35: 28–35.

Mechanic, D. (1978) 'Sex, Illness, Illness Behaviour and the Use of the Health Services', *Social Science and Medicine*, 12B: 207–14.

Meltzer, H., Gill, B., Petticrew, M. and Hinds, K. (1995) *OPCS Surveys of Psychiatric Morbidity in Great Britain: Report No. 1 The Prevalence of Psychiatric Morbidity Among Adults Living in Private Households*, London: HMSO.

Miller, R. (1993) 'The Criminalization of the Mentally Ill: Does Dangerousness Take Precedence Over Need For Treatment?', *Criminal Behaviour and Mental Health*, 3: 241–50.

Mookherjee, H. (1997) 'Marital Status, Gender, and Perception of Well-Being', *The Journal of Social Psychology*, 137: 95–105.

Morgan, M. (1980) 'Marital Status, Health, Illness and Service Use', *Social Science and Medicine*, 14: 633–43.

NAO (National Audit Office) (1989) *Financial Management in the NHS*, HC 566, London: HMSO.

Nathanson, C. (1977) 'Sex, Illness and Medical Care: A Review of Data, Theory and Method', *Social Science and Medicine*, 11: 13–25.

Oakley, A. (1984) *The Captured Womb: A History of the Medical Care of Pregnant Women*, Oxford: Basil Blackwell.

Oakley, A. (1993) *Women Medicine and Health*, Edinburgh: Edinburgh University Press.

O'Dowd, T. and Jewell, D. (eds) (1998) *Men's Health*, Oxford: Oxford University Press.

OECD (Organisation for Economic Co-operation and Development) (1996) *Health Care Reform: The Will to Change*, Paris: OECD.

OECD (Organisation for Economic Co-operation and Development) (1998) *Maintaining Prosperity in an Ageing Society*, Paris: OECD.

ONS (Office for National Statistics) (1997) *Results from the General Household Survey 1995*, London: HMSO.

ONS (Office for National Statistics) (1998) *Results from the General Household Survey 1996*, London: HMSO.

ONS (Office for National Statistics) (2000a) *Population Trends*, London: The Stationary Office, Spring.

ONS (Office for National Statistics) (2000b) *Social Trends*, London: The Stationary Office, Volume 30.

OPCS (Office of Population Censuses and Surveys) (1994) *Living in Britain: Results from the General Household Survey 1992*, London: HMSO.

OPCS (Office of Population Censuses and Surveys) (1996) *Living in Britain: Results from the General Household Survey 1994*, London: HMSO.

Parker, G. (2000) 'The Royal Commission on Long Term Care for the Elderly: New Vision or More of the Same for Social Care Policy?', in H. Dean, R. Sykes, and R. Woods (eds) *Social Policy Review 12*, Newcastle: Social Policy Association, pp. 133–56.

Parker, G. and Clarke, H. (1997) 'Will You Still Need Me, Will You Still Feed Me? – Paying for Care in Old Age', *Social Policy and Administration*, 31(2): 119–35.

Parry-Jones, W. (1972) *The Trade in Lunacy*, London: Routledge & Kegan Paul.

Payne, S. (1995) 'The Rationing of Psychiatric Beds: Changing Trends in Sex-Ratios in Admission to Psychiatric Hospital', *Health and Social Care in the Community*, 3(5): 289–300.

Payne, S. (1996) 'Masculinity and the Redundant Male: Explaining the Increasing Incarceration of Young Men', *Social and Legal Studies*, 5(2): 159–78.

Perls, T. (1997) 'Acute Care Costs of the Oldest Old', *Hospital Practice*, 32(7): 123–37.

Pfeiffer, S., O'Malley, D. and Short, S. (1996) 'Factors Associated With the Outcome of Adults Treated in Psychiatric Hospitals: A Synthesis of Findings', *Psychiatric Services*, 47(3): 263–9.

Phillipson, C. (1998) *Reconstructing Old Age: New Agendas in Social Theory and Practice*, London: Sage.

Pilowsky, L., O'Sullivan, G., Ramana, R., Palazidou, E. and Moodley, P. (eds) (1991) Women and Mental Health, *British Journal of Psychiatry*, 158: Supplement 10.

Pleck, J. (1981) *The Myth of Masculinity*, Cambridge, MA: MIT Press.

Porter, R. (1987) *Mind Forg'd Manacles: A History of Madness in England from the Restoration*, London: Athlone.

Powell, E. (1961) Speech by the Minister for Health in *Report of the Annual Conference of the National Association for Mental Health*, London: NAMH.

Power, C. (1994) 'Health and Social Inequality in Europe', *British Medical Journal*, 308: 1153–6.

Prior, P.M. (1993) *Mental Health and Politics in Northern Ireland*, Aldershot: Avebury Press.

Prior, P.M. (1999) *Gender and Mental Health*, London: Macmillan/New York: NYUP.

Prior, P.M. and Hayes, B.C. (2001a) 'Gender Trends in Occupancy Rates in Mental Health Beds in Northern Ireland', *Social Science and Medicine*, 52: 537–45.

Prior, P.M. and Hayes, B.C. (2001b) 'Changing Places: Men Replace Women in Mental Health Beds in Britain', *Social Policy and Administration*, 35(4): 397–410.

Prior, P.M. and Hayes, B.C. (2001c) 'Marital Status and Bed Occupancy in Health and Social Care Facilities in the UK', *Public Health*, 115: 401–6.

Prior, P.M. and Hayes B.C. (2002) 'Marital Status and the Use of Health and Social Care Facilities in Britain', *Journal of Family Issues*. (Forthcoming).

Ranade, W. (1994) *A Future for the NHS: Health Care in the 1990s*, London: Longman.

Regier, D., Farmer, M., Rae, D., Myers, J., Kramer, M., Robins, L., George, L., Karno, M. and Locke, B. (1993) 'One Month of Prevalence of Mental Disorders in the USA and Sociodemographic Characteristics: The Epidemiologic Catchment Area Study', *Acta Psychiatrica Scandinavica*, 88: 35–47.

Reicher-Rossler, A. and Rossler, W. (1993) 'Compulsory Admission of Psychiatric Patients – An International Comparison (Review Article)', *Acta Psychiatrica Scandinavica*, 87: 231–6.

Ribbe, M., Ljunggren, G., Steel, K., Topinkoba, E., Hawes, C., Ikegami, N., Henrard, J.C. and Jonnson, P. (1997) 'Nursing Homes in 10 Nations: A Comparison Between Countries and Settings', *Age and Ageing*, 26 (Suppl. 2): 3–12.

Roberts, H. (ed.) (1992) *Women's Health Matters*, London: Routledge.

Robins, L. and Regier, D. (eds) (1991) *Psychiatric Disorders in America: The Epidemiologic Catchment Area Study*, New York: The Free Press.

Robinson, R. and Le Grand, J. (1994) *Evaluating the NHS Reforms*, Newbury: Policy Journals.

Saigh, P. (1988) 'Anxiety, Depression and Assertion Across Alternating Intervals of Stress', *Journal of Abnormal Psychology*, 97: 338–41.

Sanguineti, V., Samuel, S., Schwartz, S. and Robeson, M. (1996) 'Retrospective Study of 2,200 Involuntary Psychiatric Admissions and Re-admissions', *American Journal of Psychiatry*, 153(3): 392–6.

Sartorius, N., Nielson, J. and Stomgren, E. (1989) 'Changes in Frequency of Mental Disorder over Time: Results of Repeated Surveys of Mental Disorders in the General Population, *Acta Psychiatrica Scandivavica*, 79 (Supplement 348).

Scheper-Hughes, N. (2001) *Saints, Scholars and Schizophrenics: Mental Illness in the Republic of Ireland*, Berkeley and Los Angeles: University of California Press.

Scull, A. (ed) (1991) *The Asylum as Utopia: W.A.F. Browne and the Mid Nineteenth Century Consolidation of Psychiatry*, London: Tavistock/Routledge.

Shapiro, E. and Tate, R. (1988) 'Who Is Really at Risk of Institutionalization?', *The Gerontologist*, 28: 237–45.

Shapiro, S., Skinner, E., and Kessler, L. (1984) 'Utilization of Health and Mental Health services: Three Epidemiologic Catchment Area Sites', *Archives of General Psychiatry*, 41: 971–8.

Shorter, E. (1990) 'Mania, Hysteria and Gender in Lower Austria 1891–1905', *History of Psychiatry*, 1: 3–31.

Showalter, E. (1987) *The Female Malady: Women, Madness and English Culture 1830–1980*, London: Virago Press. (First published 1985)

SSI (NI) (1998) *Key Indicators of Personal Social Services for Northern Ireland, A Report from the Social Services Inspectorate*, Belfast: DHSS.

Sutherland Report (1999) *With Respect To Old Age: A Report by the Royal Commission on Long Term Care*, London: HMSO.

Thomas, C., Stone, K., Osborn, M., Thomas, P. and Fisher, M. (1993) 'Psychiatric Morbidity and Compulsory Admission Among UK-Born Europeans, Afro-Caribbeans and Asians in Central Manchester', *British Journal of Psychiatry*, 163: 91–9.

Thornley, C., Walton, V., Romans-Clarkson, S., Herbison, G. and Mullen, P. (1991) 'Screening for Psychiatric Morbidity in Men and Women', *The New Zealand Medical Journal*, 104(925): 505–7.

Townsend, P., Davidson, N. and Whitehead, M. (1992) *Inequalities in Health*, rev. edn, Harmondsworth: Penguin. (First published 1988)

Ussher, J. (1991) *Women's Madness: Mysogyny or Mental Illness?*, London: Harvester Wheatsheaf.

Verbrugge, L. (1979) 'Marital Status and Health', *Journal of Marriage and the Family*, 41: 267–85.

Verbrugge, L. (1989) 'The Twain Meet: Empirical Explanations of Sex Differences in Health and Mortality, *Journal of Health and Social Behaviour*, 30: 282–304.

Verhaak, P. (1993) 'Analysis of Referrals of Mental Health Problems by General Practitioners', *British Journal of General Practice*, 43: 203–8.

Waldron, I. (1976) 'Why do Women Live Longer than Men?', *Social Science and Medicine*, 10: 349–62.

Waldron, I. (1997) 'What do we Know about Causes of Sex Differences in Mortality: A Review of the Literature', in P. Conrad (ed) *The Sociology of*

Health and Illness: Critical Perspectives, 5th edn, New York: St. Martin's Press, pp. 42–55.

Waldron, I. (2000) 'Trends in Gender Differences in Mortality', in E. Annandale and K. Hunt (eds) *Gender Inequalities in Health*, Buckingham: Open University Press, pp. 150–81.

Waldron, I., Hughes, M. and Brooks, T. (1996) 'Marriage Protection and Marriage Selection – Prospective Evidence for Reciprocal Effects of Marital Status and Health', *Social Science and Medicine*, 43: 113–23.

Waldron, I., Weiss, C. and Hughes, M. (1997) 'Marital Status Effects on Health: Are There Differences Between Never Married Women and Divorced and Separated Women?', *Social Science and Medicine*, 45: 1387–97.

Walsh, D. and Kendler, K. (1995) 'The Prevalence of Schizophrenia in Ireland: Re-assessing the Enigma', *Archives of General Psychiatry*, 52: 509.

Walters, V. (1993) 'Stress, Anxiety and Depression: Women's Accounts of Their Health Problems', *Social Science and Medicine*, 36(4): 393–402.

Watkins, T.R. and Callicutt, J.W. (eds) (1997) *Mental Health Policy and Practice Today*, Thousand Oaks, California, USA: Sage.

WHO (World Health Organization) (1946) *Constitution: Basic Documents*, Geneva: WHO.

Wilkinson, G. (1989) 'Referrals from General Practitioners to Psychiatrists and Paramedical Mental Health Professionals', *British Journal of Psychiatry*, 154: 72–6.

Wilkinson, R. (1996) *Unhealthy Societies: The Afflictions of Inequality*, London: Routledge.

Wilson, G. (2000) *Understanding Old Age: Critical and Global Perspectives*, London: Sage.

Wistow, G., Knapp, M., Hardy, B. and Allen, C. (1994) *Social Care in a Mixed Economy*, Buckingham: Open University Press.

Woolf, S.H., Joans, S. and Lawrence, R.S. (eds) (1996) *Health Promotion and Disease Prevention in Clinical Practice*, Baltimore, MD: Williams & Wilkins.

Wyke, S. and Ford, G. (1992) 'Competing Explanations for Associations between Marital Status and Health', *Social Science and Medicine*, 34: 523–32.

Zerbe, K. (1995) 'Anxiety Disorders in Women', *Bulletin of the Menninger Clinic*, 59(2): Suppl. A: A38–A52

Zlotnick, C., Shea, T., Pilkonis, P., Elkin, I. and Ryan, C. (1996) 'Gender, Type of Treatment, Dysfunctional Attitudes, Social Support, Life Events and Depressive Symptoms over Naturalistic Follow-Up', *American Journal of Psychiatry*, 153(8): 1021–7.

Author Index

Subject Index

Note: f = figure, n = note, t = table.